Advanced Nursing Practice
Second edition

Advanced Nursing Practice
Second edition

Edited by

Paula McGee and George Castledine

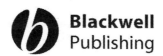

© 1998, 2003 by Blackwell Publishing Ltd

Editorial offices:
Blackwell Publishing Ltd, 9600 Garsington Road, Oxford OX4 2DQ, UK
    Tel: +44 (0)1865 776868
Blackwell Publishing Inc., 350 Main Street, Malden, MA 02148-5020, USA
    Tel: +1 781 388 8250
Blackwell Publishing Asia Pty Ltd, 550 Swanston Street, Carlton, Victoria 3053, Australia
    Tel: +61 (0)3 8359 1011

First edition published 1998
Second edition published 2003

Library of Congress Cataloging-in-Publication Data
is available

ISBN 1-4051-0234-9

A catalogue record for this title is available from the British Library

Set in 10/12.5pt Palatino
by DP Photosetting, Aylesbury, Bucks
Printed and bound in Great Britain using acid-free paper
by TJ International Ltd, Padstow, Cornwall

For further information on Blackwell Publishing, visit our website:
www.blackwellpublishing.com

Contents

Preface

This second edition of *Advanced Nursing Practice* has been extensively revised in the light of the many new opportunities created by changes in both the clinical field and health policy reforms. These changes have occurred on a global scale as part of a World Health Organisation agenda to increase access to health services by enhancing the contribution of nursing. Nurses in over 30 countries, and in diverse settings, are currently exploring new ways of meeting local health needs. In support of these developments the International Council of Nurses has developed a broad definition of advanced practice that recognises universal characteristics whilst leaving each country free to develop nursing services that best suit its needs.

This book examines the concept of advanced practice in the UK and shows how much it has developed in recent years. The advent of advanced practice, coupled with radical health service reforms has enabled senior and experienced nurses to develop and refine new clinical roles that share three key characteristics: professional maturity, the ability to challenge professional boundaries and to pioneer innovations. These characteristics form the basis of a definition of advanced nursing practice, developed by the editors, that is used, by different contributors to this book to examine the following issues:

- The forms of clinical and professional competence, based on uni-professional and multi-professional perspectives, required at this level.
- The relationship between advanced practice and clinical governance, for example through benchmarking, and the advanced practitioner's role in facilitating best, evidence-based practice through transformational leadership coupled with a high level of interpersonal competence.
- The nature of practice in the UK's multicultural society through advanced assessment and the provision of health promotion.
- The impact of advanced practice in the wider arena of healthcare especially with regard to the interface between advanced nursing and other professions, notably medicine, and the legal implications of new levels of practice.
- The possibilities for advanced practice inherent in current and future developments.

Paula McGee
University of Central England, Birmingham

Contributors

George Castledine, Professor and Consultant in General Nursing, Faculty of Health and Community Care, University of Central England and The Dudley Group of Hospitals NHS Trust.

Ann Close, Director of Nursing, Dudley Group of Hospitals NHS Trust.

Sarah Coleman, Adult Branch Curriculum Coordinator/Senior Lecturer in Evidence-based Practice, Department of Nursing and Midwifery, University College Worcester.

Bridgit Dimond, Emeritus Professor, University of Glamorgan.

Brian Ellis, Consultant Urological Surgeon, Department of Urology, Ashford Hospital, Middlesex. Director of Surgery, Ashford and St Peter's Hospitals NHS Trust. Honorary Senior Clinical Research Fellow, St Mary's Hospital, London.

Jane Fox, formerly Head of Department of Nursing and Midwifery, Department of Health, University College Worcester.

Alison Gidlow, Advanced Nurse Practitioner (Urology), The Royal Free Hospital, London.

Dean Holyoake, Advanced Nurse Practitioner in Mental Health, Priory Healthcare Adolescent Mental Health Services.

Chris Inman, Senior Lecturer and Course Leader, MSc Advanced Practice, Faculty of Health and Community Care, University of Central England.

Paula McGee, Professor, School of Health and Policy Studies, Faculty of Health and Community Care, University of Central England, and Chair, Transcultural Nursing and Healthcare Association, UK.

Trish Mason, Director of Operations and Executive Nurse, Royal Shrewsbury Hospital NHS Trust and Princess Royal Telford NHS Trust.

Abi Masterson, Director, Abi Masterson Consulting Ltd, Southampton. Abi Masterson Consulting undertakes work on new role development and evaluation for a wide range of healthcare organisations.

Peter Matthews, former Pharmaceutical Advisor, Sandwell Health Authority, West Midlands.

Lindsay Mitchell, Director, Prime Research and Development Ltd, Harrogate.

Chapter 1

Introduction

Paula McGee and George Castledine

The changing context of advanced practice

The United Kingdom Central Council (UKCC 1994: 20) defined advanced practice as 'adjusting the boundaries for the development of future practice, pioneering and developing new roles responsive to changing needs and with advancing clinical practice, research and education enrich professional practice as a whole'. This definition was part of the first attempt to clarify the nature of practice beyond initial registration and arose from the recognition that the complexity of modern health-care placed new demands on nurses, requiring them to extend their scope of practice. It also provided many opportunities to develop new roles or take on responsibilities that were undreamt of by earlier generations of the profession. These changes posed particular challenges for the Council in ensuring that developments were focused on nursing practice and, for the first time, in developing criteria against which practice beyond initial registration might be assessed and regulated.

When we prepared the first edition of this book the idea of advanced practice in the UK was new and it was not clear how, or even if, the Council's definition would translate into the realities of nurses' work. We therefore set out to examine advanced practice from the perspectives of nurses working in innovative roles in settings as diverse as learning disabilities, dementia care and cardiology. Nurses working in these fields described their practice in which they integrated multiple activities such as consultancy, education and research. In so doing these practitioners demonstrated that, regardless of the setting, they had well-developed interpersonal skills, provided coaching and guidance, clinical and professional leadership and acted as consultants for both their nursing colleagues and other professionals. We compared the work of these nurses with that of advanced practitioners in the USA whom we had invited to describe their roles. Comparison revealed many similarities in practice leading us to argue 'that some forms of nursing transcend specialisation, even though they may be based in it. There is something beyond the possession of high levels of knowledge and expertise which enables the individual practitioner to function in a different way' (McGee 1998: 177).

At the time this was as far as we felt able to go. Our research had revealed widespread confusion at senior levels in the NHS about the nature of advanced nursing roles. This research also identified concerns about the impact on patient care, possible elitism and questions about the expense of employing nurses on senior grades when it was not at all clear whether or how they differed from other practitioners (McGee *et al.* 1996). Further research indicated that this situation had begun to change with distinctions being made between advanced and other roles. A small number of NHS trusts developed specific criteria for advanced posts and expected postholders to exercise high levels of autonomy and leadership in clinical practice, to develop new roles and use their creativity in pioneering new ideas (McGee & Castledine 1999). However, some degree of confusion remained, particularly in differentiating between advanced and other roles, especially those of nurse practitioners. In response to this confusion and continued concerns about the desirability of advanced and other roles, the UKCC began a project examining nursing roles and proposed the concept of *higher-level practice* with recommendations for new and specific criteria for assessing individual practitioners (UKCC 2002).

The Council's report has now been presented to the new Nursing and Midwifery Council (NMC), the body that must consider the recommendations in the light of proposed changes in professional regulation and control. These proposed changes are intended first to simplify the professional Register by reducing it to three sections: nursing, midwifery and public health. Second, the changes aim to ensure that the Register must reflect the needs of modern society by ensuring that registrants are both professionally and personally fit to practise, consideration of which must include that required for advanced practice. The Council will have to determine whether to record all *higher-level* qualifications and what additional requirements may be needed to regulate the practice of nurses working in advanced roles at the frontiers of nursing (NMC 2002).

The work on higher-level practice took place alongside radical reforms of the health service. These were aimed at reducing health inequalities by improving both access to and the quality of healthcare by, for example, involving service users in service design and delivery and tailoring services to meet local needs (DoH 1997, 2000). In addition to broad reforms, practice must now be based on sound evidence. The National Institute for Clinical Excellence (NICE) provides authoritative guidance on best practice with regard to health technologies, the medical management of specific conditions and surgical procedures. The object is to promote quality care across the UK. NICE also has a role to play in encouraging a blame-free culture in the workplace so that poor or inappropriate practice can be challenged and professionals enabled to learn from mistakes (NICE 2003).

This climate of professional and clinical change has created many new opportunities for advanced nurses who are able to creatively combine traditional nursing expertise with new health knowledge and technologies. Such combinations exemplify the growing confidence of advanced nurses in testing out and adopting new roles even if these mean performing activities that have traditionally been the preserve of other professions. This means that advanced nurses are able to expand their practice and contribute to the development and enhancement of patient care in ways that transcend traditional professional boundaries. Advanced nurses are not becoming doctors by another name but there remain concerns both within and outside the profession as to whether their practice truly represents an advance for nursing. There are also fears that nurses may be leaving behind their legitimate work in a rush to take on tasks that they regard as more prestigious or exciting. The plethora of job titles has not helped since these give no indication as to whether the individual is practising nursing at or beyond the level of registration or some other professional role.

In view of the changes outlined here and the continuing uncertainty about advanced practice, we considered it appropriate to reconsider our ideas. The outcome is this new edition in which we assert that:

- There exists, irrespective of the terminology used, forms of nursing practice that are more than that achieved by initial registration and which are distinguishable by definable characteristics. Our term for these forms is *advanced nursing practice*
- Clarification of these definable characteristics across different fields of nursing is an essential part of:
  o legitimising advanced nursing practice and ensuring parity with other health service professionals
  o demonstrating the contribution made by advanced nursing practice to both individual patient care and the provision of a modern health service
  o developing appropriate career paths, including the academic and clinical preparation required for advanced nurse practitioners.

Key features of this new edition

This second edition of *Advanced Nursing Practice* has been extensively revised in line with current literature and research. Each chapter ends with a list of key questions that we hope will provide a basis for further discussion of, and research into, the issues raised in the chapter. In Chapter 2, George Castledine sets the scene for the book by explaining the historical development of advanced nursing practice in the UK from the perspective of a nurse who took an active part in events. This chapter is unique in that it brings together disparate elements that are not always easily accessible, to provide a comprehensive account that introduces the reader to the thinking under-pinning advanced practice. The account also demonstrates that advanced practice has not developed in a predictable or linear fashion. There have been numerous ideas and experiments, sometimes competing with or contradicting one another, but all have in some way contributed to professional discourse on the nature of nursing after regis-tration in the UK.

In Chapter 3 we present our current views on the nature of advanced nursing practice. This is based on a combination of our recent professional experience as consultants working in NHS trusts, our own research activities, involvement with the UKCC's work on higher-level practice and consideration of contemporary issues that affect advanced nursing. These issues include current health policy and the intro-duction of nurse consultant and modern matron roles. We propose our own definition of advanced nursing practice that we regard as having three key elements: professional maturity, challenging professional boundaries and pioneering innovations. We discuss our ideas for each element and clarify the competences that we regard as essential for practice at this level.

The next group of four chapters deal with competence, standards and education in advanced nursing practice. In Chapter 4, Abi Masterson and Lindsay Mitchell examine the concept of competence in nursing, arguing that this can be viewed from two perspectives: uni-professional and multi-professional. Both of these are relevant to advanced practice. Uni-professional competence is that determined by the nursing profession. The Royal College of Nursing's work on nurse practitioners and the College's faculty project on emergency nursing are used as examples to illustrate ways in which nurses themselves have identified different categories and assessment of competence beyond initial registration. In contrast, multi-professional competence is that determined by non-nurses that impacts on health professionals in general. Examples in this category include the work of the Sector Skills Council in developing occupational standards in public health and the potential impact of the Agenda for Change initiative (NHS Executive 1999). The authors of this chapter take the view that both types of competence are relevant to advanced nursing practice. The introduction of clinical governance and user involvement in service delivery means that health professionals must be open about the nature and extent of their competence not only in their own professional spheres but also in their capacity to work together.

In Chapter 5, Sarah Coleman and Jane Fox continue the focus on standards by examining clinical benchmarking. They begin by contextualising this within the debate on how best to determine and measure standards in nursing care. They argue that clinical benchmarking provides the tools for nurses to evaluate the qualitative as well as the quantitative aspects of their work. Advanced practitioners have a vital role to play in this activity by acting as a resource and consultant to colleagues, identifying and promoting best practice both within their own practice settings and in the wider professional arena. Achieving best practice based on sound evidence requires, as Ann Close argues in Chapter 6, a transformational leader with a high level of interpersonal competence and an ability to inspire others to work together. The effective advanced practitioner is able to provide clinical and professional leadership at different levels within the organisation, empowering not only those responsible for delivering direct care but also impacting on organisational policy at local and national levels.

The range of competences required in advanced nursing practice raises the question of how nurses can prepare to undertake this role. In Chapter 7, Chris Inman presents one approach to this matter in describing the master's course at the University of Central England. This course is unusual in having compulsory practice and research dissertation elements. Students are required to undertake a double module in advanced health assessment and then apply their learning to patients or clients in their own practice setting. This requirement means that students must be based in practice rather than education or management and have two practice-based facilitators who can support the development of advanced health assessment skills and role development. The focus on practice places considerable demands on students and facilitators alike. It is also a major attraction, reassuring both aspiring advanced practitioners and seconding employers that practice is valued as a core element and that successful graduates are competent to undertake their new roles.

The following four chapters concentrate on practice. In Chapter 8 Paula McGee uses a case study to clarify the differences between assessment in professional practice and that undertaken by the advanced nurse practitioner. She argues that advanced health assessment is characterised by a holistic approach in which extensive clinical knowledge is synthesised with the individual patient's story and physical data to formulate diagnoses and initiate treatment where appropriate. Advanced health assessment provides a total health database that can provide a foundation for both the monitoring of general health and the management of ongoing health problems such as asthma. In Chapter 9, Dean Holyoake presents an account of his experiences in conducting advanced health assessments. He draws on practice-based examples to argue that the therapeutic use of self is a constant factor in mental health assessments at any level but that the advanced practitioner travels a journey with the patient, from assessment to discharge, exploring with that person the experience of their illness and working with them to achieve a client-centred strategy aimed at resolving or managing that experience.

In Chapter 10, Ann Close takes a different approach in focusing initially on the expanded concept of health that informs advanced health assessment and then linking this with health promotion. She uses case studies to argue that advanced practice provides considerable opportunity for health promotion at different levels in healthcare. The advanced practitioner can work with individual clients or communities, coaching and guiding them to become better informed and take an active role in promoting or maintaining their own health. Similar work can be undertaken with local practitioners enabling them to identify opportunities for health promotion and to develop strategies for empowering their patients. At more senior levels, advanced practitioners can apply their skills in research to identify specific health issues requiring attention, initiate health promotion strategies and influence policy. Finally, in Chapter 11, Paula McGee examines advanced practice within the context of the UK's multicultural society and the health inequalities experienced by many members of minority ethnic groups. She argues that advanced practitioners have an important role to play as change agents, combating institutional racism and ensuring that services are accessible, sensitive and responsive to local needs.

The final group of chapters addresses a broad range of issues in advanced nursing practice. In Chapter 12, Paula McGee presents an international perspective situating advanced practice within a global agenda for nursing as defined by the World Health Organisation (WHO 2000). The potential of advanced nursing practice is currently being explored in at least 30 countries, in all continents, with diverse health needs and varying levels of wealth. Whilst nurses in the USA have made the most progress in both theoretical and practice development, their counterparts in Ireland, Fiji and many other countries are making steady progress, focusing on marrying the WHO agenda with the healthcare needs of their own populations. Their efforts are now supported by a definition and set of competences for advanced practice published by the International Council of Nurses (ICN 2002).

Some of the issues raised in Chapter 12 are then discussed within the context of the UK. First is the interface between advanced nursing practice and medical practice. We have already stated that advanced practitioners are not trying to take over medical work, but there are indications that some of our medical colleagues experience unease about the development of advanced nursing roles. In Chapter 13, Alison Gidlow, an advanced practitioner, and Brian Ellis, a medical consultant, clarify the distinctive differences between their two roles, arguing that the traditionally pre-eminent position of medicine is challenged by the complexity of patient needs and the current emphasis on multidisciplinary working. Inherent in this challenge is the potential for true collaboration based on equality and valuing the expertise of different health professionals. Moreover, patients recognise the benefits of consulting practitioners who have more time to spend with them. The way forward lies in transparency in which medical and nursing staff jointly support the development of advanced nursing roles and in which new initiatives are subject to robust evaluation.

Allied to the interface with medicine is the authority of the advanced nurse practitioner to initiate treatment. Inevitably this raises questions about the right to prescribe medication. In Chapter 14, Peter Matthews, a pharmacist, outlines the background to and policy underpinning the introduction of nurse prescribing. He argues that a combination of factors has contributed to change: a growing population of elderly people, the continual development of drug technology and increased public expectations. Moreover, the farcical practice that required competent nurses, able to make decisions about prescribing, to ask a doctor to write a prescription, clearly needed to be challenged. Enabling nurses to prescribe in their own right is consistent with current policy about increasing access to healthcare and frees up doctors' time for other activities. The preparation and assessment of nurses for such responsibility is clearly important and raises a number of legal as well as professional issues.

The prescription of medicines is only one aspect of advanced practice that has legal dimensions. As Bridgit Dimond points out in Chapter 15, there are so many legal issues, including human rights, accountability, delegation and supervision and patients' rights, that they could form the sole topic for a book. However, in summing up her arguments she states that individual practitioners, at whatever level they function, remain personally and professionally accountable for their practice and must ensure that they are competent to perform the activities required in their field. They are also responsible for ensuring that they maintain their competence and that there is appropriate supervision of those activities that they delegate to others.

A final dimension of the issues raised in Chapter 11 is the political context in which advanced practice is developing. In Chapter 16 George Castledine argues that nurses often shy away from politics because they either cannot see the point of becoming involved or they lack the skills required to do so. As this chapter shows, the development of nursing continues to be contingent upon the exercise of political acumen by individuals and professional organisations. Advanced practitioners are in positions in which they can shape the future of nursing care by engaging in political activities and using political processes for the benefit of their patients. They can do the same in lobbying for a career path and appropriate conditions of service. In Chapter 17, Trish Mason and George Castledine present an account of work undertaken in Shrewsbury and Telford hospitals on clarifying advanced roles. They then apply this as a basis for proposing a clinical career structure.

In Chapter 18 we draw the book to a close by emphasising the importance of retaining a focus on nursing in advanced practice rather than allowing practitioners to be absorbed into the junior practice of medicine. In so doing we recognise that we are presenting a challenge to advanced nurses to creatively express nursing values, knowledge and skills in hitherto uncharted territory. Despite the advances made since the first edition of this book was published, we recognise that there is still much to be done, particularly in relation to employment and career development, if advanced nursing practice is to become fully established. Moreover, in the continuously changing environment of the health service we recognise that there will always be new initiatives that offer more opportunities. One example is the development of first contact services. Currently in the pilot stage, these services could provide useful professional and political leverage for astute advanced practitioners to provide articulate leadership in nursing. We recognise that research is vital in determining the success of these initiatives and in evaluating the impact of advanced practice on patient care. We therefore present an agenda that we hope will stimulate the interest of researchers and act as a catalyst for future investigations.

References

DoH (Department of Health) (1997) *The New NHS: Modern, Dependable*. London: DoH.

DoH (Department of Health) (2000) *The NHS Plan: A Plan for Investment, A Plan for Reform*. Wetherby: DoH.

ICN (2002) http://www.icn.ch (accessed September 2002).

McGee, P. (1998) Advanced practice in the UK. In: *Advanced and Specialist Nursing Practice* (Eds G. Castledine & P. McGee), pp. 177–84. Oxford: Blackwell Science.

McGee, P. & Castledine, G. (1999) A survey of specialist and advanced nursing practice in the UK. *British Journal of Nursing*, **8** (16): 1074–8.

McGee, P., Castledine, G. & Brown, R. (1996) A survey of specialist and advanced nursing practice in England. *British Journal of Nursing*, **5** (11): 682–6.

NHS Executive (1999) *Agenda for Change – Modernising the NHS Pay System. Joint Framework of Principles and Agreed Statement on the Way Forward*, HSC 1999/227. Available at http://www.doh.gov.uk

NICE (2003) available at http://www.nice.org.uk

NMC (2002) available at http://www.nmc-uk.org

UKCC (1994) *The Future of Professional Practice – The Council's Standards for Education and Practice following Registration*. London: UKCC.

UKCC (2002) *Report of the Higher Level of Practice Pilot and Project*. London: UKCC.

WHO (2000) *Global Advisory Group on Nursing and Midwifery, Report of the 6th Meeting*. Geneva: WHO. Available at www.who.org (accessed September 2002).

Chapter 2

The Development of Advanced Nursing Practice in the UK

George Castledine

Introduction

The history of advanced nursing practice in the UK is fragmentary and poorly documented[1] but available evidence suggests that, alongside the development of clinical nurse specialist roles during the 1970s, grew the idea that some nurses were capable of even more demanding activities (Ashworth 1975). The nature of these activities was not then clear but a number of experimental appointments were made. For example, Gillie (1975) pointed out that a new, consultant nurse role could be developed to fill the gap created by a shortage of junior doctors. Millington (1976) actually worked as a nurse consultant in anaesthetics and found that a large part of her work involved pre- and postoperative counselling and dealing with problems related to equipment and techniques. Other appointments were made in child health. However, there appears to be an absence of research into and evaluation of these consultant appointments and so it is difficult to determine the extent of their contribution; it is not certain how they differed from clinical nurse specialist roles or how they might relate to modern nurse consultants (Castledine 1998a). Often, terms such as advanced, specialist and consultant were used synonymously during the 1980s and early 1990s to refer to levels of practice beyond initial registration, which serves to further confuse the situation. What persisted over time was the idea of a level of

---

[1] Particularly when compared with specialist nursing as discussed by Castledine (1998a, b) in the first edition of this book.

practice that differed from that of the nurse specialist. This chapter presents an account of the disparate influences and ideas that have helped to shape the current concept of advanced practice.

The Post-registration Education and Practice Project

The initiation of Project 2000 in the 1980s and subsequent reforms in nurse education added to the professional debate about levels of practice and the need to look towards a practitioner-centred division of labour to provide flexibility at a time of rapid change. The registered practitioner needed support from those with additional experience and education; thus simply working in a speciality was not a sufficient basis for the expertise that the provision of such support required. The climate of change in the practice setting and reform in education provided a timely opportunity for a review of post-registration practice in nursing. This was commissioned by the United Kingdom Central Council (UKCC) which emphasised the importance of combining experience with formal education because only those practitioners 'who have advanced their knowledge and skills through education and experience can exercise increasing clinical discretion and accept greater professional responsibility through advanced practice' (UKCC 1991). In the final report the Council endorsed two concepts of practice development following registration as a nurse: specialist and advanced.

Specialist practice was defined as a type of specialised clinical role that required the nurse to 'exercise the highest levels of judgement and discretion in clinical care ... demonstrate higher levels of clinical decision making ... monitor and improve standards of care through supervision of practice, clinical nursing audit, developing and leading practice, contributing to research, teaching and supporting professional colleagues' (UKCC 1994: 9). In contrast, advanced practice involved 'adjusting the boundaries for the development of future practice, pioneering and developing new roles responsive to changing needs and, with advancing clinical practice, research and education, to enrich professional practice as a whole' (UKCC 1994: 20). The development and achievement of both these forms of nursing practice was dependent not only on those individuals working in such roles but also to a great extent on the active support of NHS trust managers. In the year following the publication of the Council's report, a survey of 230 NHS trusts in England, which between them claimed to employ nearly 2500 specialist nurses, showed that the most common fields of practice for such individuals was in the physical dimensions of care that reflected medical specialities. There were far fewer advanced practitioners (n = 119), but these also were employed mainly in physical care. Job descriptions, where they existed, were invariably non-standard, tailored to individuals in particular posts in specific areas with little commonality between them even in the same trust. The grading of posts, employment conditions, work activities and concerns about the interface between advanced practice and medicine all emerged as matters requiring attention. Added to this was a lack of understanding, among senior managers, regarding the differences between specialist and advanced nurse practitioners (McGee *et al.* 1996).

A further survey of 283 NHS trusts across the UK showed a continued lack of differentiation between specialist and advanced roles compounded by the increasing numbers of nurse practitioners. The number of trusts employing advanced practitioners was now 36.2% but still much lower than those employing specialist nurses (87%). The focus on physical care was upheld, although mental health was now included in the most common fields of practice. There was an emergent consensus that advanced nurses engaged primarily in clinical practice that differed from that of specialist nurses. Advanced practitioners were expected to conduct advanced assessments, make referrals, conduct their own clinics, order investigations, prescribe, and treat minor injuries. They also provided leadership and were a source of advice for patients, staff and other professionals locally, regionally and nationally on a much greater scale than specialist nurses. However, they undertook teaching and research in much the same way as specialist nurses (McGee & Castledine 1999).

Castledine's criteria for advanced practice

The report of the Post-registration Education and Practice Project pointed out that advanced nursing practice was not to be regarded as an additional tier of nursing practice. In other words, the advanced practitioner was not simply an extension to the specialist role in which the nurse becomes even more knowledgeable and adept. Rather, advanced practice is a distinct sphere of nursing (UKCC 1994). This suggested that the clinical career ladder to advanced practice did not necessarily have to be through specialist practice, thus encouraging those nurses who worked in a more general field of nursing or across medical specialities to develop their nursing care at an advanced level. It will be interesting to see in the future if such 'generalist' advanced practitioners develop and reach fruition.

This view of advanced practice as independent from the specialist role led Castledine (1996) to propose specific criteria, roles and functions of advanced nurse practitioners as it was developing in the UK in the mid-1990s. These were broken down into seven categories (Fig. 2.1).

Autonomous practitioner
Experienced and knowledgeable
Researcher and evaluator of care
Expert in health and nursing assessment
Expert in case management
Consultant, educator and leader
Respected and recognised by others in the profession

Fig. 2.1 Key criteria of an advanced nursing practitioner.

(1) *Autonomous practitioner.* Advanced nurse practitioners (ANPs) should be resourceful enough to work on their own, contributing to either one or more multidisciplinary healthcare teams and perhaps linking institutional care with community and home-based care.

(2) *Experienced and knowledgeable.* ANPs should be expert in a particular field of nursing that may be closely linked to a specialist area of medicine or other related subject. They should have at least eight years' post-registration experience. Some may have worked as a specialist nurse practitioner but they must all have a sound theoretical and practical knowledge of nursing and the medical or other area that is related to their practice. This level of knowledge should be at master's degree and be relevant to their work.

(3) *Researcher and evaluator of care.* One of the key areas for ANPs is conducting research and evaluation into various areas of their work. They should be able to utilise nursing theory and research in order to analyse problems. A good understanding of quality assurance and audit is important.

(4) *Expert in health and nursing assessment.* ANPs should be able to conduct a comprehensive health and nursing assessment when working with patients, and be particularly skilled in the holistic aspects of patient assessment. At the same time, they must be able to narrow down their focus to the patient's particular medical and/or health concern, identifying the differences between nursing and medical approaches to health assessment.

(5) *Expert in case management.* The emphasis of the ANP role should be on case management treatment of complex problems/concerns that are within the individual practitioner's domain and responsibility. The focus of the ANP should be the effects of disease or disability on the patient and/or family. Furthermore, the ANP should be working with the patient and/or family to enable the achievement of a productive lifestyle or peaceful death.

(6) *Consultant, educator and leader.* ANPs must act as consultants and educators in all matters relating to their chosen field and role. For this reason, ANPs should be good communicators, change agents and leaders of nursing. There will be times when they will teach not only patients and families but also nurses, doctors and other members of the healthcare service.

(7) *Role model.* ANPs must be respected and recognised by their colleagues as authorities in their particular field. Such recognition only comes with time and the publication of their work.

Many nurses feared that a very heavy medical orientation would be imposed on the ANP role, particularly as a result of recent changes in junior doctors' hours and the shortages of medical staff. Consequently, Castledine (1996) emphasised the importance of advanced clinical nursing practice being guided by a nursing model and not be directed or dictated by physicians or a medical model. He also stressed that the educational preparation of the ANP of the future should be a clinically based master's degree built on the criteria in Fig. 2.1.

Government intervention

The strategy for nursing launched in 1999 outlined the development of a new career structure for nurses (DoH 1999). This structure consisted of four career bands, starting with healthcare assistants and cadets, and rising to a top band, comprising consultant nurses and those working at a 'higher level of practice'. It was Prime Minister Tony Blair who had announced a year early in 1998 that he wanted to see the introduction of nurse consultant posts. There was no formal piloting of the new concept, and without adequate funding the roles were slow to develop. The purpose behind the posts was to help provide better outcomes for patients by improving services and quality, to strengthen leadership and to provide a new career opportunity to help retain experienced and expert nurses, midwives and health visitors in practice. The Department of Health (DoH 1999) outlined four core functions of the consultant posts:

- An expert practice function
- A professional leadership and consultancy function
- An education, training and development function
- A practice and service development research and evaluation function

It was strongly recommended that all consultant nurse posts should be firmly based in practice with at least half the working time spent in direct contact with patients, clients or communities (DoH 1999). To support the academic and research side of the role it was further hoped that many of the posts would establish formal links with local universities. NHS organisations were invited to submit proposals for one or two posts and include evidence shown in Table 2.1. It was hoped that those nurses

Table 2.1 The evidence required from NHS bodies with regard to appointing consultant nurses (DoH 1999).

- Plans are based on a thorough needs assessment, that they are consistent with government policy and clearly designed to benefit patients, clients or communities
- The purpose and responsibilities of the post are clearly specified and the post invested with professional and organisational autonomy and authority commensurate with its intended purpose
- The professional competences needed have been identified and that arrangements have been made to establish that candidates meet these requirements
- An assessment of risks and professional and legal liability has been made and appropriate indemnification planned or arranged
- The role is clearly located in the wider healthcare team, enabling the postholder to complement and work collaboratively with others
- Any substitution for medical, technical or other roles does not obscure professional accountability for the fundamental nursing, midwifery and health visiting function at the core of the consultant role
- The postholder will be properly supported and have opportunities for continuing professional development
- Arrangements are planned or in place to monitor the contribution made and to enable adjustments to be made to the post to maximise benefits and minimise risks

working at consultant/higher level would typically have been educated and trained to master's or doctorate level, hold professional registration and additional specialist-specific professional qualifications.

The government suggested that the skills and competences necessary for nurse consultant postholders should be developed according to the UKCC's recommendations for higher-level practice (UKCC 1999). However, it also pointed out that although the government supported the Council's work, not all those who were accredited as working at a higher level of practice would necessarily become consultant nurses (NHS Management Executive 1999). The criteria for appointment would depend more on the employer's view of the practitioner's ability, role and contribution to the local service. In effect, the Department of Health's regional offices carefully controlled the whole process of appointment to consultant posts.

Towards a higher level of practice

Rapid changes in healthcare, the reduction in junior doctors' hours, the advent of new clinical roles such as nurse practitioners, the rise in specialist nurses and the move of post-registration education into higher education led the Council to re-examine its post-registration framework. In August 1997, a specialist practice task group was established to consider how the existing framework for specialist practitioners could embrace nurse practitioners, clinical nurse specialists and advanced practitioners. Later, in 1998, this group, now called the Higher Level Practice Steering Group, was charged with the task of recognising and clarifying possible levels of practice, in particular, one at a higher level.

The group examined the competences and the assessment criteria needed to engage in higher levels of practice. The framework that emerged was tested on consumers, the profession and stakeholders through a series of national consultation events. This resulted in the identification of the specific outcomes against which practitioners could be assessed and the design of a robust assessment system. A report of this consultation was circulated to individuals and organisations, including patient groups, service managers, academic heads, the national boards for nursing in the UK, government health departments and representatives of other health and social care professions. The report was well received and the Higher Level Practice Steering Group was directed by the Council to carry out a pilot study to test how well the competences and assessment framework could be used in practice.

The pilot ran from November 1999 to March 2001. Almost 700 nurses, midwives and health visitors volunteered to take part as either candidates or members of assessment panels. The methods of investigation included completion of a special profile, interview by a panel, questionnaires and visits to the candidates' workplace. The conclusion of all this work was reported to the June 2001 UKCC council meeting in Glasgow. It showed that it is possible to articulate a standard for higher-level practice and, although some modifications will be needed, the standard, which involves a series of seven domains, can be used as a basis for identifying nurses and midwives working at a higher level of practice.

The higher-level practice standard and assessment system set the context for the development of initiatives such as nurse and midwife consultants. Many employers used it to structure job descriptions, to inform lifelong learning and to support risk management. The standard was a significant step in recognising nurses and midwives who have stayed in the clinical area and have achieved an advanced level of practice. The term 'higher-level practice' was intended as only a temporary term, not meant to remain after the work of the UKCC had been completed. Castledine (2002) therefore urged the new Nursing and Midwifery Council to revert to using the terms 'advanced practice' and 'advanced practitioner'. Such a move was encouraged because it fitted in with international developments in other countries such as Ireland, Australia, the USA and Canada.

Advanced nursing practitioners

Very few nurses and midwives are officially recognised as working at the level of advanced practice. One of the reasons for this is the amount of experience that seems to be required to develop appropriate expertise. In a study reported in Chapter 17 of this book, Castledine and Mason found that, out of 50 nurse specialists in the NHS hospital trust, there were only 6–8 nurses truly working at a higher level. It would seem that considerable experience, approximately 10 years, is needed before the full development of specific competences for advanced practice can be realised.

Castledine and Mason argue that, using the same principles developed by the UKCC for higher-level practice, criteria for all clinical nurses, especially those working in specialist practice, could be identified. This would means that it is the 'level' of responsibility, functioning and competence that will determine how individuals are recognised, rather than the title they are using. For example, just because someone uses the title 'nurse practitioner' or 'nurse specialist' it does not mean that they are working at a higher level than an experienced staff nurse. What is now clearly emerging in British nursing is the need to recognise, accept and adopt levels of clinical practice, with the first one starting immediately on qualifying and the last one finishing with higher-level practice. The recognition of levels would provide a much clearer clinical career framework or structure.

Job titles

The job titles nurses use should reflect the levels of responsibility and functioning inherent in their roles. The trouble is that there are numerous job titles being used by nurses throughout the UK and their proliferation has led to confusion not only among patients but also within the profession itself. Titles appear to be used by nurses as a means of conveying some type of status or authority. Often titles are handed out or adopted because no one can be bothered to identify the specific competences, knowledge and skills that are inherent in a particular role. The increasing emphasis on a competence-based approach from student nurse preparation onwards is now helping to clarify the specific aspects of a nurse's job. If we can achieve that, we should be able to standardise nursing titles at all levels, thus avoiding all the present confusion and misunderstanding.

Conclusion

This chapter has outlined the major historical features of advanced practice, highlighting some of the early attempts to develop roles beyond initial registration. In contrast to specialist nursing these early attempts were poorly documented and reflect the absence of an established programme of research. More recent developments at national level have been recorded, for example by the UKCC, but there remains an absence of research at local levels. Too often roles are introduced without evaluation of their effectiveness or sharing of the lessons learned with those beyond the immediate setting (McGee & Castledine 1999). There is an urgent need for the systematic recording and evaluating of existing and emergent advanced roles as well as research that examines the potential contributions of advanced to future healthcare.

This chapter has also shown that, whilst there was initially some professional pressure for these roles, it has been the joint efforts of the UK government and UKCC that have led the way in establishing a model for advanced practice and outlining the criteria and content of standards. Much continues to be done to promote and develop clinical leaders but what is needed most are those dynamic senior professionals who so often in the past have been keen to question nursing and the future direction of the profession. Healthcare professionals have been called upon to re-examine their practices, professional values and beliefs about the delivery and outcomes of healthcare. There is an emphasis on cross-boundary working and new working practices that sweep away old-fashioned interprofessional demarcations. The government of 2003 wants nurses and other healthcare professionals to take on new technical medical roles, and in the case of nursing, to shed traditional nursing care practices. It is in this arena that advanced practice will continue to develop, led by those nurses who are prepared, through practice and education, to expand the horizons of the profession to meet the healthcare needs of the new century. In taking up this challenge we invite you to consider the key questions set out below.

 Key questions for Chapter 2

In your field of practice:

(1) In what ways does current health policy challenge professional values, beliefs and practices?
(2) What are the characteristics of advanced nursing roles?
(3) What arrangements are or can be made for documenting the setting up, progress and evaluation of new or experimental nursing roles in your workplace?

References

Ashworth, P. (1975) The clinical nurse consultant. *Nursing Times*, 17 (15): 574–7.

Castledine, G. (1996) The role and criteria of an advanced nurse practitioner. *British Journal of Nursing*, 5 (5): 288–9.

Castledine, G. (1998a) Clinical specialists in nursing in the UK: the early years. In: *Advanced and Specialist Nursing Practice* (eds G. Castledine & P. McGee), pp. 3–32. Oxford: Blackwell Science.

Castledine, G. (1998b) Clinical specialists in nursing in the UK: 1980s to the present day. In: *Advanced and Specialist Nursing Practice* (eds G. Castledine & P. McGee), pp. 33–54. Oxford: Blackwell Science.

Castledine, G. (2002) Higher Level Practice is in fact Advanced Practice. *British Journal of Nursing*, 11 (7): 1166.

DoH (1999) *Making a Difference: Strengthening the Nursing, Midwifery and Health Visiting Contribution to Health and Healthcare*. London: DoH.

Gillie, O. (1975) Plan for nurse consultants to fill doctor gap. *Sunday Times*, 14 September.

McGee, P. & Castledine, G. (1999) A survey of specialist and advanced nursing practice in the UK. *British Journal of Nursing*, 8 (16): 1074–8.

McGee, P., Castledine, G. & Brown, R. (1996) A survey of specialist and advanced nursing in England. *British Journal of Nursing*, 5 (11): 682–6.

Millington, C. (1976) Clinical nurse consultant in anaesthetics. *Nursing Mirror*, 142 (20): 49–50.

NHS Management Executive (1999) *Nurse, Midwife and Health Visitor Consultants*, HSC 1999/217. London: NHS Management Executive.

UKCC (1991) *The Report of the Post-registration Education and Practice Project*. London: UKCC.

UKCC (1994) *The Future of Professional Practice – The Council's Standards of Education and Practice following Registration*. London: UKCC.

UKCC (1999) *A Higher Level of Practice. Report on the Consultation on the UKCC's Proposals for a Revised Regulatory Framework for Post-registration Clinical Practice*. London: UKCC.

UKCC (2002) *Report of the Higher Level of Practice Pilot and Project*. London: UKCC.

Chapter 3

A Definition of Advanced Practice for the UK

Paula McGee and George Castledine

Introduction

The United Kingdom Central Council (UKCC) first used the term 'advanced practice' formally in its report on post-registration education and practice (UKCC 1994). In some ways this report represented the culmination of years of development in which individual nurses explored the possibilities inherent in their work and experimented with new ideas that seemed both to meet patients' needs and to provide meaningful professional activity. The result was a patchwork of established and emergent nursing roles beyond initial registration that the Council sought to streamline. Alternatively, the report on post-registration education and practice can be seen as a beginning of a thorough examination, by the nursing profession, of the nature of practice after registration and how this could best meet the needs of patients. This examination encouraged considerable and useful debate and research as well as – perhaps inevitably – rather a lot of confusion. The lack of certainty posed challenges for many professionals, including tutorial staff on courses that prepared nurses to become specialist or advanced practitioners. One of those challenges was to be able to answer questions from students and non-nursing staff, about the nature of advanced practice, in appropriate and meaningful ways. Another was to present advanced practice to health service managers who had responsibility for making decisions about the need for this level of nursing and whether they should send staff onto courses.

This chapter begins by examining some of the issues in advanced practice. This is followed by the authors' definition of advanced practice that has been developed in response to a perceived need to articulate the unique characteristics of this form of nursing in both educational and practice settings. This definition is discussed and represented as a model that provides nurses and members of other disciplines with a framework for understanding the contribution that advanced practitioners can make to patient care and service delivery.

Influences on advanced practice in the UK

The United Kingdom Central Council

One of the principal influences on advanced practice has been the work of the United Kingdom Central Council, which defined advanced practice as:

> adjusting the boundaries for the development of future practice, pioneering and developing new roles responsive to changing needs and with advancing clinical practice, research and education enrich professional practice as a whole. (UKCC 1994: 20)

At the time it was not clear how this definition would apply to the reality of daily life. Consequently, the number and range of posts and roles continued to grow without any formal check or scrutiny. McGee and Castledine's (1998, 1999) survey of NHS trusts throughout the UK found that advanced nurses were employed in 60 different fields of practice with the most common being accident and emergency, night duty, mental health and ophthalmology. How many of these nurses conformed to the UKCC's (1994) definition of advanced practice was unclear. Senior nurses in 14% ($n = 280$) of NHS trusts either did not or could not differentiate between specialist and advanced roles and only three trusts were able to provide criteria for appointing advanced nurses.

Despite these shortcomings there emerged an acceptance that practice was not static and that nursing must continue to move forward even if the direction in which it should do so was not entirely clear. There was also agreement that formal preparation, beyond the level of initial registration, was a necessity and that advanced practice should contain a clinical component that included advanced assessments, ordering diagnostic tests, treating patients and referring them to other sources of help as well as acting as a source of professional advice to colleagues (McGee & Castledine 1998, 1999; Wilson-Barnett *et al.* 2000).

There was additional confusion about the interface between advanced nurses and nurse practitioner roles that were introduced as part of a series of initiatives to reduce junior doctors' hours following the publication of the New Deal (NHS Management Executive 1991) by the Department of Health (DoH). There was no overall plan regarding nurse practitioner roles and consequently several parallel developments took place. For example, in many instances, nurses taking over tasks previously performed by doctors were awarded the title of nurse practitioner even though they had received minimal preparation for the work in comparison with others who had undertaken postgraduate study. A survey of the North Thames Region identified four categories of nurse practitioner: nurses who performed specified procedures, those in charge of pre-admission clinics, designated posts in accident and emergency departments or minor injuries units, and nurses who had extended their skills in order to perform certain tasks for their caseload of patients (Kendall *et al.* 1997). In contrast, a study in primary care showed nurse practitioners acting as the first point of contact with the health service and thus having assessment and diagnostic responsibilities similar to prototype nurse practitioner roles in the 1980s (Burke-Masters 1986; Stillwell *et al.* 1987; Ashburner *et al.* 1997).

The Royal College of Nursing

The Royal College of Nursing developed a definition of the nurse practitioner role that has now been expanded and updated to take account of that issued by the International Council of Nurses (ICN 2002). The College defined a nurse practitioner as 'a registered nurse who has undertaken a specific course of study of at least first degree (honours) level and who fulfils specified criteria' (RCN 2002) – see Table 3.1. The College identified seven domains for nurse practitioner practice. These were based on those of the American National Organisation of Nurse Practitioner Faculties (NONPF) see Table 3.2. Each domain was accompanied by a set of competences to be achieved. For example, the nurse–patient relationship had ten competences that included creating a climate of mutual trust, maintaining confidentiality and bringing the relationship to an end (RCN 2002). The College is currently in the process of developing a NONPF forum in the UK and held an inaugural meeting for interested parties in November 2002. If the profession accepts

Table 3.1 Royal College of Nursing criteria for nurse practitioner roles (RCN 2002).

A nurse practitioner is one who:

- Makes professionally autonomous decisions, for which she/he is accountable
- Receives patients with undifferentiated and undiagnosed problems and makes an assessment of their healthcare needs based on highly developed nursing knowledge and skills including skills not usually exercised by nurses such as physical examination
- Screens patients for disease risk factors and early signs of illness
- Makes differential diagnosis using decision-making and problem-solving skills
- Develops with the patients an ongoing nursing care plan with an emphasis on preventative measures
- Orders necessary investigations and provides treatment and care both individually as part of a team and through referral to other agencies
- Has a supportive role in helping people to manage and live with illness
- Provides counselling and health education
- Has the authority to admit or discharge patients from their caseload and refer patients to other healthcare providers as appropriate
- Works collaboratively with other healthcare professionals
- Provides leadership and consultancy as required.

Table 3.2   Domains for nurse practitioner practice (RCN 2002).

- Management of patient health/illness
- The nurse–patient relationship
- The teaching coaching function
- Professional role
- Managing and negotiating healthcare systems
- Monitoring and ensuring the quality of healthcare practice
- Cultural competence

these competences and domains, then appropriately prepared nurse practitioners may be recognised as advanced practitioners.

Higher-level practice project

In an attempt to resolve the uncertainty and confusion surrounding advanced practice, the UKCC began a process of consultation with practitioners and stakeholders that demonstrated support for the concept of higher-level practice (UKCC 1999) – see Table 3.3. According to the Council, higher-level practitioners were able to apply their extensive knowledge, experience, wisdom and skills to develop practice and improve care for patients. Colleagues and patients regarded them as experts in their fields. They were professionally mature and able to exercise a high level of critical judgement. Following this consultation, the Council pressed forward with a pilot scheme to develop and test a standard for higher-level practice. The standard was then tested throughout the UK via assessment of individual practitioners and upheld with some modifications (UKCC 2002). The outcomes were referred to the newly constituted Nursing and Midwifery Council when it replaced the UKCC and a response is currently awaited.

Expert practice

One of the issues arising from the introduction of higher-level practice is the apparent conflation of 'expert' and 'higher-level' practice. This is compounded by the decision

Table 3.3   Outcomes of the UKCC's consultation on higher-level practice.

- 97% of respondents ($n = 2023$) supported the idea that aspiring higher-level practitioners should be registered
- 92% agreed that such practitioners should notify the UKCC at regular intervals of their intention to practise
- 91% supported the idea that aspiring higher-level practitioners should have practised for a specified period before being assessed
- 89% supported the idea that aspiring higher-level practitioners should spend the majority of their time in practice
- 78% supported the idea of signifying a higher-level practitioner by the letter H, but responses were inconclusive as to what else should be recorded, e.g. degrees and other non-professional qualifications
- 68% supported the idea that aspiring higher-level practitioners should have a degree relevant to their field

to award all those participants in the Council's pilot scheme who were deemed to meet the higher-level standard the status of advanced practitioners. Thus the concepts of expert, higher-level practice and advanced practice appear to have become inter-changeable without any formal consideration. A brief trawl through the research-based literature raises questions about the wisdom of this. First there is the notion of expert identified by Benner (1984) as the pinnacle of nursing. In her view, the expert nurse is one who is no longer rule-bound, has extensive experience, and is highly proficient and capable of fluid, flexible performance. The expert nurse 'has an intuitive grasp of each situation and zeroes in on the accurate region of the problem without wasteful consideration of a large range of unfruitful, alternative diagnoses and solutions' (Benner 1984: 32). In other words, what makes expert nurses different from others is their ability to intuit the fundamental characteristics of a situation by clearing away irrelevant information. This notion of the intuitive grasp reflects the phenomenological approach used in Benner's (1984) study and is concerned chiefly with clinical performance. The seven dimensions of the standard for higher-level practice acknowledge the importance of clinical care but also address other issues such as improving quality and health outcomes, leadership and innovation (UKCC 1999). Similarly, Hamric (2000) argues that clinical performance is central to advanced practice but that the practitioner must also demonstrate competence in other domains such as ethics and collaboration. Thus the idea of expert clinical performance is part of but not the whole of advanced and higher-level practice.

In contrast, Jasper's (1994) analysis of the concept of expert identifies four attributes. The expert must possess a specialised body of knowledge and extensive experience beyond that expected in other practitioners and be able to use this to generate new knowledge. However, the nature and extent of this knowledge and experience is vague so that 'although experts may be able to share their knowledge it may not be possible to define what it is or predict what it may be in the future' (Jasper 1994: 772). This dubious position implies that expert knowledge cannot be clearly articulated. If this is the case then there is no way of knowing whether or how expert knowledge differs from that of others. There may also be no way of knowing how nurses acquire such knowledge and whether mandatory academic study to become higher-level or advanced practitioners is worth the effort.

Knowledge and experience provide a framework for pattern recognition. This enables experts to identify similar clinical situations in diverse settings (Jasper 1994). The expert takes a holistic view of a situation, focusing on what is most important rather than details, acting with enthusiasm because whilst situations may be similar, each one is encountered for the first time (Zukav 1979; Jasper 1994). This analysis lends some credence to Oberle and Allen's (2001: 151) argument that expert knowledge 'is largely experientially acquired whereas the APN [advanced practice nurse] has a greater store of theoretical knowledge acquired through graduate study'. This combination of theoretical and experiential knowledge equips the advanced practitioner to study the unknown and act as a generator for new knowledge. In scientific terms, the expert may be equated to a technician who is 'a highly trained person whose job is to apply known techniques and principles. He deals with the known', whereas the advanced practitioner, like a scientist 'deals with the unknown' (Zukav 1979: 36). If this is the case then the knowledge base for higher-level practice requires some scrutiny before it can be equated with that of advanced practice.

Finally, Jasper (1994) argues that experts are acknowledged by other people, peers deemed qualified to make judgements about the quality of an individual's work. This is also a feature of the UKCC's definition of higher-level practice. Advanced practice also requires recognition by others. For example, Hamric (2000) proposes that one of the core competences for advanced practice is that of acting as a consultant, providing advice for other nurses and non-nursing professionals. Meeting the requirements of this competence is dependent upon recognition by others that the individual possesses specialist knowledge and skills outside their domain (Barron & White 2000). Some form of public acknowledgement is, therefore, a shared feature of expert, higher-level and advanced practice. In advanced practice this recognition is largely based on assessment during academic study and relationships with co-professionals. Higher-level practice also requires a detailed and formal assessment by peers, but recognition of experts may be far less rigorous and therefore open to challenge.

Health policy and reform

An additional sphere of influence on advanced practice is health policies and reforms instigated by the Labour government during the late 1990s and early 2000s. These were intended to improve the quality of services by ensuring that they were tailored to meet local needs and reduce health inequalities (Table 3.4). The reforms were also aimed at valuing staff and developing a more transparent approach to both the management of information and the decision-making process (DoH 1997, 2000, 2001a). The strategy for nursing that accompanied the introduction of these policies and reforms made clear that the profession had an essential role to play because it was seen as ideally placed to promote health, particularly in community settings such as schools and places of work (Table 3.5). Nurses' skills and expertise could be directed towards early identification and treatment of health problems and the provision of support for those with chronic conditions, especially during periods of crisis. Such nurse-led activity could offset the need for more expensive services, including admission to hospital. Where such admission was necessary, nurses could use their

Table 3.4   Core principles of current health policy and reforms (DoH 1997, 2000, 2001a).

- Provision of a universal service based on clinical need and available to all
- Provision of a comprehensive range of services
- Services tailored to meet the needs of individuals, families and carers which includes seeking their views/participation
- Response to the needs of different populations
- Continuous effort to improve the quality of services and minimise errors
- Support and value staff
- Funds for healthcare devoted solely to NHS patients
- Collaboration with others to ensure a seamless service
- Promote health and reduce health inequalities
- Respect confidentiality of individuals and provide open access to information about services, treatment and performance

Table 3.5 The role of nursing in current health reforms (DoH 1999).

- Promoting health particularly in the community – healthy schools, workplaces and neighbourhoods – and with socially excluded populations
- Providing faster access to services, for example through NHS Direct, walk-in centres and other nurse-led initiatives
- Enabling people to remain at home and avoid admission by acting as assessors, care coordinators, and providing specialist practice and rapid response to crises
- Prescribing medicines without referral to a doctor
- Expanding roles in acute care settings in collaboration with medical and other staff to develop care pathways, increased specialist skill and promote evidence-based practice
- Providing intermediate care and promoting independence for people with complex needs
- Tackling specific problem areas such as nosocomial infections
- Promoting seamless care and inter-agency working

skills to develop care pathways, promote continuity of care and address specific problems such as infection control (DoH 1999).

These views about nursing were shared by the British Medical Association (BMA 2002), which argued that there was a need to address how best to make use of medical skills as the demands on doctors increased and their numbers declined. The Association proposed that, in primary care, the first contact for most patients could be a nurse practitioner. This nurse could either provide an expanded range of direct care or refer the patient on to the most appropriate service that might be medical, nursing or another health profession. In hospital settings a specialist nurse could act as the care coordinator within and across care settings. This specialist nurse would also have an advanced clinical role, the nature of which would depend on the speciality. The BMA argued that these proposals would ensure better coordination of services with fewer referrals and handovers and better provision of information for patients. They could also serve to reduce complaints and litigation (BMA 2002).

Nurse consultants and modern matrons

A final influence on the development of advanced practice has been the introduction of two new senior nurse grades: nurse consultant and modern matron. Both roles were intended to bring about improvements in the delivery of care. The matron roles were introduced following public consultation that revealed a preference for the presence of a clearly identified clinical leader, in hospital settings, who could remedy shortcomings in the service. Matrons were to take charge of groups of wards to provide leadership and direction for staff and maintain a visible and authoritative presence to whom patients and families could turn for support (DoH 2001b). These matrons were to be part of the system of nursing management. However, a study of senior nurses in one north London NHS trust found that trying to separate specialist and managerial roles was far from clear-cut because ward managers often perceived themselves as having specialist expertise (Williams *et al.* 2001). Managerial status may even confer benefits in terms of access to formal power structures and authority to initiate activities. The focus of advanced practice means that practitioners generally do not have managerial status, but the question then arises as to whether having a separate role is in any way a hindrance, and research is needed to examine this issue.

In contrast to the matrons, nurse consultants were to be clinical leaders of frontline nursing staff in both hospital and community settings, but free from the demands of managerial responsibilities (Ashworth 1975). They were to be expert practitioners who spent at least half their working time in practice working directly with patients and empowering nurses, midwives and health visitors by acting as focal points for professional advice, education and research – activities similar to those required by advanced practitioners. Their posts were to provide opportunities for experienced and skilled practitioners to remain in practice rather than have to move into management or education to further their careers (DoH 1999; 2001c). Reports indicated that consultant and matron roles could complement one another. For example, Dewing and Brooks (2002) described their joint work in arguing that their different roles enabled them to develop a shared vision and to support, rather than rival, each other.

The introduction of matron and consultant roles alongside those of nurse practitioners, specialist nurses and others may indicate that, as in the USA, advanced practice is an umbrella term for those who have undergone a specified preparation and met identified criteria. However, the emergent nature of all these roles militates against this in the short term. The UKCC's work provided a beginning but it must be recognised that roles are likely to undergo changes as they develop: 'testing the water', 'learning to swim' and 'heading for shore' (Stern 1985).

'Testing the water' is an exploratory stage in which both practitioners and managers assess the practice settings to ascertain current strengths and weaknesses, build the foundation of good working relationships with colleagues and begin to identify ways in which the new role may contribute to improvements. From this exploration will emerge an initial role that is subsequently refined by 'learning to swim'. At this stage various versions and aspects of the role can be tried out to see which best meet the demands of the setting. With such experience comes recognition of what works, what does not and why. A key element of this stage is regular dialogue between those involved. Such dialogue should also include legal advice and appraisal by employers, their legal advisors and insurers, of the vicarious liabilities involved. Finally, in 'heading for shore' the new role becomes better established but requires regular review as practitioners, managers and advisors develop a clearer understanding of the role.

The next section of this chapter takes account of the issues discussed here and presents the authors' views on advanced practice.

Conceptualising advanced practice

Our argument about advanced practice is based on our experience as consultants in NHS trusts, working with the UKCC on higher-level practice and on our research. In our view, advanced nursing practice is *a state of professional maturity in which the individual demonstrates a level of integrated knowledge, skill and competence that challenges the accepted boundaries of practice and pioneers new developments in healthcare.* The key

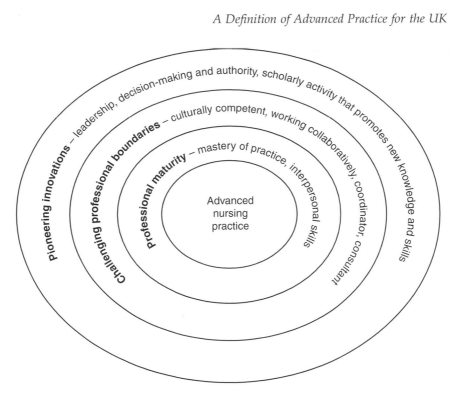

Fig. 3.1   The key elements of advanced nursing practice.

elements inherent in advanced nursing practice are set out in Fig. 3.1 and examined in greater detail below.

Professional maturity

We first take the view that the advanced practitioner should have practised in a wide range of settings and with diverse client groups in order to generate the experiential database that is fundamental to expert clinical performance. This database is complemented by interpersonal skills that enable the advanced practitioner to identify the individual patient's preferred style of communication and adapt accordingly to ensure meaningful and effective exchanges. Inability to provide effective care or to communicate disqualifies the individual from advanced practice. The experiential database is enhanced by and integrated with theoretical knowledge acquired through formal study yielding a recognised academic qualification at postgraduate level. This synthesis of two different ways of knowing enables the advanced practitioner to engage 'in a dialectic between the general and the particular' (Oberle & Allen 2001: 152), in which theoretical and experiential knowledge are brought together with knowledge of the characteristics of the particular patient. New possibilities emerge based on a refined understanding of the situation and the outcomes desired.

In our view, formal qualifications are an essential part of establishing the credibility of the advanced practitioner among a peer group drawn from other disciplines. In addition, the advanced practitioner holds a senior position in the organisation. Our own surveys demonstrated that whilst the majority of advanced practitioner posts were graded at G or H, a small number, 6% (n = 102), were at F or E. A total of 75% of trusts (n = 283) had no policy on the grading of advanced practitioner posts (McGee & Castledine 1999). We take the view that appointing advanced practitioners to posts with low grades makes it difficult for those individuals to function in a health service that is still predominantly hierarchical in nature. Thus senior positions are important in enabling advanced practitioners to have the power and authority needed to fulfil their roles and at the same time be regarded as equals by their colleagues. Thus, in our view, the advanced practitioner is one who has achieved professional maturity through a synthesis of experience and formal study, works alongside senior colleagues in other disciplines as an equal and who is able to apply the insight gained in caring for, and interacting with, patients with multiple and complex needs.

Challenging professional boundaries

We next take the view that modern healthcare requires members of all professions to work in collaboration since no one discipline can meet all the needs of patients. Collaboration is an interpersonal process based on a shared sense of purpose and respect for the expertise of colleagues. It requires a willingness to share problems and the ability to communicate both effectively and constructively (Hanson *et al.* 2000). Collaboration does not require everyone to agree, but it does enable professionals to consider differing perspectives and solutions and broaden their views of what can be done to help patients. Despite these benefits, collaboration can be difficult to achieve especially as part of developing new roles. One reason for this is the different philosophies of care adopted by the various professions. Notions of confidentiality, for instance, may differ considerably and hamper the sharing of information (Conlon 1997). A second reason is the ways in which members of other professions conceptualise nursing. McGee and Ashford (1996) in a survey of nurses' and podiatrists' knowledge of each other's roles, found that each had limited understanding of the other's potential contribution to care. For example, 13% (n = 113) of podiatrists did not know that nurses could administer intravenous drugs. The advanced practitioner needs to be astute in educating fellow professionals about the possibilities inherent in this new role and demonstrate creative leadership in promoting collaborative styles of working in which nursing expertise is valued and referred to as a source of advice and help.

Creative leadership requires cultural competence, a continuous process of development in which the individual strives towards working effectively within the cultural context of the individual or community (Campinha-Bacote 1996). In this context, cultural competence refers to the interaction of self-awareness, organisational knowledge and the application of skills. The advanced practitioner is interpersonally competent, able to recognise the preferred styles of communication within an organisation and adapt either to make effective use of these existing strategies or to introduce new, more appropriate channels in ways that suit the setting. This interpersonal competence complements the advanced practitioner's understanding of the organisation and how it operates; how staff members perceive each other, relationships between staff and managers, organisational procedures and receptivity to change (McGee 1998). In becoming culturally competent the advanced practitioner is able to challenge the status quo and introduce new perspectives in a constructive manner. Thus, in our view, the advanced practitioner challenges the boundaries of practice by working collaboratively with others in ways that both enhance patient care and demonstrate to fellow professionals the possibilities of the role.

Pioneering innovations

We take the view that the advanced practitioner engages in critical practice, that is an open-minded and reflective approach to providing care (Brechin 2000). Critical practice is, therefore, rooted in respect for others. There are three elements to this type of practice (Fig. 3.2). Critical analysis is directed towards the evaluation of the patient's situation and professional interventions. The application of critical reflective skills enables the practitioner to engage in different levels of analysis which may be immediate or form the basis of ongoing inquiries. Such inquiries will not only involve dialogue with others but will also lead the practitioner into scholarly activity, such as evaluating evidence and undertaking research, that promotes the development of new professional knowledge and skills.

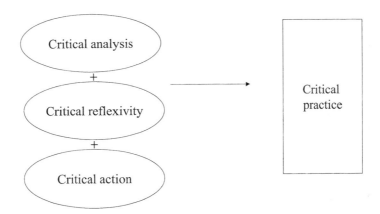

Fig. 3.2   Critical practice.

Reflection helps to identify differing perspectives on the situation and the possibility of more than one course of action. Ethical dilemmas may arise in which there is a choice of actions, all of which may be morally right but only one can be applied (Eby 2000). The advanced practitioner is able to draw on an understanding of ethical frameworks and reasoning to make decisions that are morally sound and based on respect for persons. Critical action is about the outcomes of critical analysis and reflection, the application of skills in ways that empower the recipients and avoid oppression.

Critical practice provides a basis for the advanced practitioner to act as a clinical and professional leader who identifies new and radical opportunities for nursing and acts to make these a reality even though there may be risks involved. Interpersonal competence is an essential ingredient here in communicating to others what is to be achieved and in gaining their active support and participation. Gaining and maintaining the support of others requires the ability first of all to sell them the idea and then to negotiate with them to further refine it. Providing leadership becomes part of a cooperative enterprise in which followers actively participate, catalysing their own innovations in practice. Thus in our view the advanced practitioner has a critical approach to practice through which the boundaries of nursing are examined, implemented and tested, through a synthesis of scholarly, interpersonal and reflective skills, for the benefit of patients.

Conclusion

This chapter has presented a discussion of some of the key issues in advanced practice in the UK. In particular it has sought to unravel some of the confusion over terms such as 'expert' and 'higher-level' practice that at times appear to be used interchangeably. We have argued that whilst expert practice is a part of advanced practice, it is not the whole of it. Advanced practice involves a synthesis of a wide range of knowledge and skills that are applied in specific ways to pioneer new developments in nursing. Whether advanced practice can be equated with higher-level practice is not yet clear and we have argued against the current conflation of these two terms until the relationship between the two has been further investigated. We hope that the following key questions will be helpful in furthering investigation into some of the issues we have raised here.

 Key questions for Chapter 3

In your field of practice:

(1)   What is considered to be expert practice, by whom and why?
(2)   How might the interface between advanced and other senior nurse roles be evaluated?
(3)   To what extent does our view of advanced nursing practice reflect local needs and developments?

References

Ashburner, L., Birch, K., Latimer, J. & Scrivens, E. (1997) *Nurse Practitioners in Primary Care: The Extent of Practice and Research.* Keele University, Centre for Health Planning and Management.
Ashworth, P. (1975) The clinical nurse consultant. *Nursing Times,* 17 (15): 574–7.
Baron, A. & White, P. (2000) Consultation. In: *Advanced Nursing Practice: An Integrative Approach* (eds A. Hamric, J. Spross & C. Hanson), pp. 217–44. Philadelphia: W.B. Saunders.
Benner, P. (1984) *From Novice to Expert: Excellence and Power in Clinical Nursing Practice.* Menlo Park, CA: Addison-Wesley.

BMA (2002) The future healthcare workforce, HPERU Discussion Paper 9. Available at http://www.bma.org.uk

Brechin, A., Brown, H. & Eby, M. (eds) (2000) *Critical Practice in Health and Social Care*. London: Sage/Open University.

Burke-Masters, B. (1986) The autonomous nurse practitioner: an answer to the chronic problem of primary care. *The Lancet*, 31 May, p. 1266.

Campinha-Bacote, J. (1996) A culturally-competent model of nursing management. *Surgical Services Management*, 2 (5): 22–5.

Conlon, M. (1997) The Hub in Bristol. Unpublished workshop paper presented at the Homeless and Roofless Conference, Birmingham, July.

Dewing, J. & Brooks, J. (2002) *The effects of consultant nursing practice on practice development.* Paper presented at Enhancing Practice 2: Innovation, Creativity, Patient Care and Professionalism Conference, Royal College of Nursing/Foundation of Nursing Studies, Keele, September.

DoH (1997) *The New NHS: Modern, Dependable*. London: DoH.

DoH (1999) *Making a Difference: Strengthening the Nursing, Midwifery and Health Visiting Contribution to Health and Healthcare.* London: DOH.

DoH (2000) *The NHS Plan: A Plan for Investment, A Plan for Reform.* Wetherby: DoH.

DoH (2001a) *Involving Patients and the Public in Healthcare*. Discussion Document. London: DoH. Available at www.doh.gov.uk

DoH (2001b) *Implementing the NHS Plan: Modern Matrons. Strengthening the Role of Ward Sisters and Introducing Senior Sisters*, HSC 2001/10. Available at http://www.doh.gov.uk/hsc.htm

DoH (2001c) More NHS nurse consultants. *News Desk* 10 September. Available at www.doh.gov.uk/newsdesk/archive

Eby, M. (2000) The challenge of values and ethics in practice. In: *Critical Practice in Health and Social Care* (eds A. Brechin, H. Brown & M. Eby), pp. 117–40. London: Sage/Open University.

Hamric, A. (2000) A definition of advanced nursing practice. In: *Advanced Nursing Practice: An Integrative Approach* (eds A. Hamric, J. Spross & C. Hanson), pp. 53–74. Philadelphia: W.B. Saunders.

Hanson, C., Spross, J. & Carr, D. (2000) Collaboration. In: *Advanced Nursing Practice: An Integrative Approach* (eds A. Hamric, J. Spross & C. Hanson), pp. 315–47. Philadelphia: W.B. Saunders.

ICN (2002) http://icn.org (accessed September 2002).

Jasper, M. (1994) Expert: a discussion of the implications of the concept as used in nursing. *Journal of Advanced Nursing*, 20: 769–76.

Kendall, S., Latter, S. & Rycroft-Malone, J. (1997) *Nursing's Hand in the New Deal: Nurse Practitioners and Secondary Health Care in North Thames.* Chalfont St Giles: Buckinghamshire College.

McGee, P. (1998) *Models of Nursing in Practice: A Pattern for Practical Care*. Cheltenham: Stanley Thornes.

McGee, P. & Ashford, R. (1996) Nurses' perceptions of roles in multidisciplinary teams. *Nursing Standard*, 10 (45): 34–6.

McGee, P. & Castledine, G. (1998) *A Survey of Specialist and Advanced Practice in the United Kingdom.* Birmingham: Nursing Research Unit, University of Central England.

McGee, P. & Castledine, G. (1999) A survey of specialist and advanced nursing practice in the UK. *British Journal of Nursing*, 8 (16): 1074–8.

NHS Management Executive (1991) *Junior Doctors: The New Deal*. NHSME: London.

NHS Management Executive (1999) *Nurse, Midwife and Health Visitor Consultants*, Health Service Circular 1999/217.

Oberle, K. & Allen, M. (2001) The nature of advanced nursing practice. *Nursing Outlook*, 49 (3): 148–53.

RCN (2002) *Nurse Practitioners: An RCN Guide to the Nurse Practitioner Role, Competencies and Programme Accreditation.* London: RCN.

Stern, P. (1985) Teaching transcultural care in Louisiana from the ground up. *Health Care for Women International,* 6 (1–3): 175–86.

Stillwell, B., Greenfield, S., Drury, M. & Hull, F.M. (1987) A nurse practitioner in general nursing practice: working style and pattern of consultation. *Journal of the Royal College of General Practitioners,* 37: 154–7.

UKCC (1994) *The Future of Professional Practice – The Council's Standards for Education and Practice following Registration.* London: UKCC.

UKCC (1999) *A Higher Level of Practice. Report on the Consultation on the UKCC's Proposals for a Revised Regulatory Framework for Post-registration Clinical Practice.* London: UKCC.

UKCC (2002) *Report of the Higher Level of Practice Pilot and Project.* London: UKCC.

Williams, A., McGee, P. & Bates, L. (2001) An examination of senior nurse roles: challenges for the NHS. *Journal of Clinical Nursing,* 10: 195–203.

Wilson-Barnett, J., Barribal, K.L., Reynolds, H., Jowett, S. & Ryrie, I. (2000) Recognising advanced nursing practice: evidence from two observational studies. *International Journal of Nursing Studies,* 37: 389–400.

Zukav, G. (1979) *The Dancing Wu Li Masters.* London: Rider.

Chapter 4

Developing Competences for Advanced Nursing Practice

Abi Masterson and Lindsay Mitchell

Introduction

The view of advanced practice presented in Chapter 3 emphasises the importance of competence. In the UK, and internationally, an increasing number of organisations are producing and/or using competence statements for nurses at all levels of practice. These organisations include commissioners of services, employers, professional bodies and associations such as the Royal College of Nursing, regulatory bodies, education and training providers. In this chapter we critically review such developments and consider their implications for advanced practice. We begin with a brief exploration of the concept of competence and chart the rise of the competence movement in nursing. We then review the respective roles of the RCN and the Nursing and Midwifery Council (previously the United Kingdom Central Council for Nursing, Midwifery and Health Visiting (UKCC)) in developing, assessing and monitoring competences for levels of practice beyond the point of registration. Finally we describe some multi-professional competence development initiatives that are likely to have a tremendous impact on advanced nursing practice.

The concept of competence

Competence is defined by the *Collins Cobuild Dictionary for Advanced Learners* (3rd edn, 2001) as 'the ability to do something well or effectively'. Mitchell (2000) has classified existing competence models in common use in health and social care into three broad types:

- Personal competence models – what people are like
- Educational competence models – what people need to possess
- Performance outcome models – what people need to achieve

She suggests that each of the different models have different purposes but can be used in combination.

Personal competence models

Personal competence models focus on individuals' personal qualities, skills, motives and aspirations – a mixture of characteristics that are thought to have a direct impact on both individuals' ability to perform and their willingness to do so. Personal competence models have their roots in psychology and are believed to be useful for individual and team development purposes. They are derived from identifying and analysing the characteristics of the 'best performers' as compared with those who are average or below average, i.e. they are norm-referenced. Assessment of individuals against these models may be norm-referenced (for example, whom would it be better to select for this post?), or self-referenced (for example, how much have I improved since the last time I was assessed?). Personal competence models are of limited use in assessing whether someone is fit for practice in an area of work because the assessment is not made against agreed benchmarks of practice.

Personal competence models have been widely used in the field of management to describe the characteristics of 'excellent managers' as compared with other managers, using characteristics such as judgement, self-confidence and strategic perspective. These characteristics are usually further described through the use of behavioural indicators, i.e. the behaviours that excellent performers most often demonstrate. For example, the key behaviours, which would indicate judgement, might include: 'identifies the most important issues in a complex situation, identifies new patterns and interprets events in new ways' (Management Charter Initiative 1997). The behavioural indicators provide the basis for agreeing the nature of the competence between different individuals.

As personal competence models have their roots in distinguishing the 'excellent' from the 'usual', they have tended to be used in development programmes which are individually designed or which are intended to 'cultivate' the few at the expense of the many. They are useful for self-assessment and development purposes in that they enable individuals to think through and self-assess their own strengths and weaknesses. However, one of their flaws is that they are often context-free.

The Royal College of Nursing's recent work on expertise in nursing, which is reviewed in more detail later in this chapter, appears to have used personal competence concepts to identify the distinguishing features of expert nurses from others. This initiative aims primarily to enable individual practitioners to express and articulate their competence and to gain recognition for this expertise. As a result of this process it is thought that it should be possible to develop programmes and support structures to develop such expertise in others. A potential weakness of this initiative, however, is that if the resulting model of competence is norm-referenced and based on being better than others in some way, as practice improves, the distinctions between individuals may well disappear.

Personal competence models also have an inherent tension within them relating to 'natural ability' as compared with 'the effectiveness of development'. Therefore personal competence models can, at their extreme, be criticised as being anti-education and anti-training if they are accompanied by assumptions that excellence is born and not developed. Owing to their focus on personal characteristics, it is also questionable whether they should be linked at all to any form of assessment that results in certification.

Because of their history and the basis of their development, personal competence models are more likely to apply to:

- The elite rather than the many
- Those with status and power (such as senior managers) as compared with those who have neither.

Educational competence models

Educational competence models focus on what it is that someone needs to know or be able to do by the end of a period of learning – normally termed 'learning outcomes'. The learning outcomes may be pre-set (programmes with clearly defined objectives) or individually negotiated (as in learning contracts). Such 'competence-based education and training' usually focuses on a combination of knowledge, skills, attributes and outcomes and may be informed to a greater or lesser extent by practice. The focus of these models is the development of individuals and the models have their roots in education and the social sciences. These models are particularly evident in the development of learning outcomes and modularisation in higher education. Educational competence models are usually informed by theories of development and hierarchies of skills and knowledge (such as Bloom's *Taxonomy* (1956)).

Learning outcomes have principally been developed by education and training providers to identify what an individual will be able to know and do by the end of a course of education and training. Such competence statements tend to be owned and led by educationalists. When learning outcomes are defined solely by educators, then it is possible that:

- They will reflect the interests of the individual educators concerned
- They may be constrained by the professional base of the educators concerned
- They may be related to specific types of learning and assessment opportunities (for example, those available to the particular students within that institution or on that particular type of course)

The outcomes developed by the UKCC (1999) for entry to the branch programmes (end of year 1 outcomes) and competences for entry to the Register (end of year 3 branch programmes) following the work of the Education Commission 'Fitness for

Practice', can be seen to be examples of the learning outcomes approach because they identify what nursing and midwifery pre-registration students need to achieve at different points in their education and training.

Assessment of educational competence models may be criterion-referenced. This is where a judgement is made regarding whether or not the individual has achieved the learning outcome. More usually it is based on grade-related criteria, i.e. individuals are allocated grades related to the extent to which they have developed, and can demonstrate, the knowledge, understanding and skills specified in the learning outcomes. Occasionally these models, whilst intending to be competence-based, may have spurious rating scales attached to them, or 'an authority' decrees that only a certain percentage can achieve the outcomes (i.e. a norm-referenced approach is inappropriately cast across a criterion-referenced/grade-related system).

Performance outcome models

Performance outcome models focus on the standards and criteria that anyone who undertakes a particular area of work or activity is expected to achieve. A process of consensus-forming and negotiation is usually used to set the level of expected achievement, although the level can also be informed by observation and analysis of work. The specification can focus on minimum standards of practice or good practice standards. Such models can be generic models, designed to be applied to different areas of practice, or can be aimed at particular areas of work. The competence statements may focus on the here and now and/or include emerging future requirements. These models focus on social roles and their roots are in sociology and socio-linguistics. Such models are useful for determining whether people are meeting the standards required at work and, from this, making decisions about their education and development needs. Performance outcome models usually consist of two parts: what needs to happen – the outcome that needs to be achieved – and the level – standard/criteria – at which it needs to happen, which is usually set at the level of good practice.

Employers usually define performance outcomes in consultation with employees, professional and regulatory bodies, and education and training interests. Critics have suggested that such competence statements are task-focused and reductionist and do not sufficiently reflect the complexities of professional practice. Additional concerns have been expressed about the focus on commonality, rather than differences, between professions, which does not truly reflect the unique nature of a particular profession. Others argue that performance criteria are useful for some career development stages such as entry to professions but are not of so much use for those working at more senior levels, for example senior managers, to whom personal competence approaches are more suited. Educationalists often express fears that a sole focus on the demands of work may be retrospective and limit true learning, reflection and development.

Assessment of performance outcome models is criterion-referenced with the outcomes and standards/criteria serving as the assessment criteria. The assessment is useful for determining whether people are meeting the standards required for particular areas of work. From such information it is also possible to work backwards to make decisions about their education and development needs.

National occupational standards are the most widely used form of performance outcomes in the UK. They are used as the basis of vocational education and training programmes and awards approved and accredited by the Qualifications and Curriculum Authority and the Scottish Qualifications Authority. The responsibility for developing national occupational standards lies with national training organisations (NTOs) and the currently emerging sector skills councils (SSCs). SSCs (and NTOs) are recognised and partially funded by the Department for Education and Skills to lead the development of the workforce within a particular sector of work. The emerging SSC for health is Skills for Health (previously the NTO Healthwork UK). The government has expressed a strong interest in performance outcome models. This is because performance outcome models are based on what it is that individuals need to achieve at work and help bridge the oft-perceived gap between education and practice. Such competence models enable education and training programmes to be linked directly to work and facilitate the development of credit frameworks for learning wherever it takes place and from whatever route, allowing individuals to change careers and career pathways.

Evaluating models of competence

Competence is a much used and abused term. Some organisations and individuals make erroneous claims to be using competence-based approaches when what they have done is little more than re-badge an existing approach. It is beyond the scope of this chapter to evaluate the quality of the examples of the wide range of different competences that exist in nursing and healthcare. A number of them do not directly relate to one of the models outlined above but instead combine, either by accident or design, features of the different models, sometimes to such an extent that it is difficult to ascertain exactly what the originators had in mind. Our own view is that it is necessary to be clear about the purpose of using a competence approach before deciding which model to use or whether competences need to be specifically developed.

Models of competence should probably be judged on the extent to which they serve the purposes for which they are or were intended. Boak (1998) suggests that the difference between more and less effective models lies in the relationship between three key characteristics:

- Accuracy – the model expresses the actual capabilities required for effective performance and does not omit any areas which are relevant to effective performance.
- Acceptability – the model is accepted as accurate and helpful to the people who are to use it, i.e. those whose competence it describes and those who have to work with the model. It is suggested that this relates to how far the model accords with the experiences of users, the degree of face validity of the development methodology to users and the degree to which it is in harmony with the other priorities affecting the user.
- Accessibility – the ease with which the model can be understood and applied by users.

Competence and nursing

Competence in nursing can be described from two main perspectives: a uni-professional perspective and a multi-professional perspective. This section reviews each of these in turn and considers their potential impact on the profession.

A uni-professional perspective

A number of initiatives have been undertaken to define competence in nursing and specifically at an advanced level. Some of these have been at national, or even international, level whereas others have focused on the development of local competences at organisational (trust) level. This brief review of competence development focuses on the former using examples of work undertaken by the Royal College of Nursing (RCN) and the United Kingdom Central Council (now the Nursing and Midwifery Council). However, we recognise that some useful local developments have taken place often to meet specific local needs, such as difficulties in recruiting particular types of staff.

The Royal College of Nursing

The Royal College of Nursing is a registered charity that functions both as a professional association and a trade union. It campaigns on behalf of nurses and nursing and provides a wide range of services for its members across the UK. It is founded on a Royal Charter and its activities include labour relations, professional representation, and, through the RCN Institute, the provision of higher education, professional accreditation and the promotion of research, quality and practice development. The RCN has been at the forefront of debates about advanced practice in the UK. It led the development of nurse practitioner programmes in the UK and has undertaken work into the nature of 'expert practice' and is in the process of developing post-registration competences in a number of specialities under the auspices of its Faculty Project.

The RCN's Nurse Practitioner initiative has been heavily influenced by the core competences outlined in the *Advanced Nursing Practice: Curriculum Guidelines and Program Standards for Nurse Practitioner Education* published by the National Organization of Nurse Practitioner Faculties in the USA (NONPF 1995). These core competences describe the generic practice behaviours of nurse practitioners upon entry into practice. The competencies were based on research done by Patricia Benner and Karen Bryckzynski who defined domains for advanced nursing practice (RCN 2002). The six domains are:

(1) Management of client health status
(2) The nurse–client relationship
(3) The teaching–coaching function
(4) Professional role
(5) Managing and negotiating the healthcare delivery system
(6) Monitoring and ensuring the quality of healthcare practice

These domains were developed from observation of and interviews with nurse practitioners in primary care practice and could therefore be classified as a performance outcome model although they have also been used as learning outcomes for programmes preparing nurse practitioners in primary and secondary care.

The RCN's Expert Practice Project aims to:

- Recognise and value expertise in nursing practice
- Develop a recognition process for expertise in practice
- Develop further understanding of the concept of expertise in different specialisms within UK nursing
- Explore the links between expertise and outcomes for service users and healthcare providers.

The Expert Practice Project involved volunteers from RCN Practice Forums (all RCN members have the right to belong to practice forums) who, through a supportive and developmental relationship with a critical companion, were helped to prepare evidence from their practice to demonstrate their expertise. The project worked on the premise that nurses experience difficulty in explaining the exact nature of their contribution to healthcare as their work often appears diffuse and is difficult to articulate. The project developed a model of expertise drawn from the literature to help practitioners reflect on and define their clinical ability. The model takes a personal competence approach to competence and is based on five key attributes of clinical expertise. The five attributes are designed to provide a structure against which evidence of expertise is provided from specific practice situations involving the nurse and their client/patient within any designated specialism or field of practice. In addition, factors that enable the development of expertise are also outlined and need to be demonstrated. The expertise model is summarised in Table 4.1.

Finally, the Faculty Project undertaken with the RCN's Accident and Emergency (A&E) Association was designed to develop a framework for integrating clinical practice, practice development, education, research, and policy development for emergency nurses that included an infrastructure to support accreditation and peer review, promoting standards of care and the value of clinical practice. The project identifies general core competences as well as more specific ones, and also the benchmarks of a career progression model. The intention is to develop: UK-wide standards of competence; a core educational curriculum that can be used as a template by education providers when devising their own programmes and courses; and ways in which individuals and A&E departments can be accredited for their achievements.

The RCN does not intend to be the sole or preferred supplier of educational courses and clinical competence programmes, but it seeks to define the competence levels, core curriculum and expected outcomes upon which universities or trusts will base their own programmes. The aim of the project is to develop nursing practice in a way that ensures patients receive the highest standards of care and assists nurses in achieving their own professional goals. The RCN hopes that the competences will enable employers to judge more effectively the standard of knowledge, skills and competence of potential employees and make sure that their employees receive the right support in order to develop. Managers will be able to identify the education and

Table 4.1   The expertise model (RCN 2000).

Attributes of expertise	Involving the following (examples only)
(1) Holistic practice knowledge	• Looking at all aspects of patient/user need • Appreciating that there is a whole • Understanding the impact on the client and their family
(2) Saliency – identifying the most pertinent issue for the patient/client and then acting on this appropriately	• Prioritising • Getting to the heart of the matter quickly • Being able to respond promptly to identified priorities with immediate action
(3) Knowing the patient/client	• Acknowledging the person as an individual and trying to see the world through that person's eyes – this is instinctive for the expert • Being accessible, being able to empathise and communicate in a personalised way • Forming a relationship and rapport promptly
(4) Moral agency – related to responding to the patient/client as a person – respecting their dignity, protecting their personhood in times of vulnerability, helping them to feel safe, providing comfort and maintaining integrity in the relationship	• Not being paternalistic, but respecting the individual's right to make their own choices • Advocating for the patient/client when they are unable to do this for themself • Being genuine, displaying warmth, working in partnership • Providing choice, enabling involvement
(5) Skilled know-how	• Demonstrating both interpersonal as well as technical skill • Intuitive decision-making • Ability to respond in a seamless, appropriate and holistic way
ENABLING FACTORS The characteristics which pre-empt the development of expertise in practice	• Reflective ability • Organisation of practice • Interpersonal relationships • Authority and autonomy • Recognition by others

skill needs of staff and help them achieve their potential more effectively. Nurses using the defined levels of competence will also be able to decide what their own education and career development needs are. The clinical, work-based focus is also intended to ensure that education and practice development will be relevant and applicable to working life.

An extensive analysis of existing clinical competence and curriculum documents for

A&E nursing has been undertaken. This has enabled a detailed description of the reality and challenges of contemporary A&E nursing practice. Wide-ranging work has been carried out to devise the levels of clinical competence and set the elements of a core educational curriculum. The work is being guided by steering groups of A&E nurses, managers and lecturer-practitioners in consultation with staff working in the field. Further consultation is planned with those working in higher education, the medical profession, the NMC and with more RCN members. Patient and user groups have also been asked to join the steering group. The general core competences reflect the key abilities required by nurses at each level and encompass the themes of knowledge base, nursing intervention, patient management and practice development. The specific competences are designed to cover the key abilities for nurses at the different levels in eight subjects/areas of practice relating to emergency nursing.

The approach taken by the Faculty Project combines a learning outcome model with aspects of a performance outcome model, i.e. the competences generally focus on the knowledge and skills that an individual needs to develop and how these would be assessed (Table 4.2, items 2 and 3). Some of the competences, however, are more linked to what needs to happen within the area of practice (Table 4.2, item 1).

It is worth noting here that the Faculty Project has used the term 'performance criteria' in a different way from that used in national occupational standards. This highlights one of the problems in making sense of the competence literature and in critically reviewing different competences. The Faculty Project's use of the term

Table 4.2 Competences from the RCN's Faculty Project.

Competence	Performance criteria
(1) Care for a patient receiving a bedside blood transfusion, demonstrating checking procedures, monitoring and an awareness of potential complications	OSCE; case studies relating to transfused patients; observation of practice
(2) Critically examine the important functions of nursing through the trauma nursing process and act independently within a multidisciplinary, multi-agency context	Documentation of impact of self throughout the trauma nursing process with reflection; current educational certification and reflection; literature review of current best evidence-based practice and application of findings; development of audit tools to evidence the value of the experienced trauma nurse with reflection
(3) Demonstrate an in-depth knowledge and the ability to apply pathophysiology and aetiology to a patient presenting with a complaint relating to the: • cardiopulmonary system • neurological system • renal system • immune system	Case studies demonstrating an application of physiological theory to practice; observation of practice; case studies; evaluation of case presentation; reflective diary

'performance criteria' relates to the assessment evidence that could be used to determine whether an individual demonstrates the competence or not. There are no criteria directly related to performance as such, that is to say using the term 'performance criteria' to mean 'a standard by which something is judged or evaluated'. The approach to competence used by the Faculty Project is in contrast to the performance outcomes approach taken by the UKCC in its developments related to a higher level of practice – this forms the next example.

The Nursing and Midwifery Council

Nursing, midwifery and health visiting are self-regulated professions in the UK. Professional self-regulation is a contract between the public and the nursing, midwifery and health visiting professions. It allows the professions to regulate their own members in order to protect the public from poor or unsafe professional practice. The current regulatory body is the Nursing and Midwifery Council (NMC), which was formally established in April 2002 and has four fundamental functions:

• Keeping the Register of members admitted to practice
• Determining standards of education and training for admission to practice
• Giving guidance about standards of conduct and performance
• Administering procedures, including making rules, relating to misconduct, unfitness to practice and similar matters

In addition, the Council may record in the Register marks indicative of competence in a field or at a level of practice. These include competences beyond what is required for registration if deemed necessary for public protection purposes.

Discussions around post-registration regulation have been a perennial feature of the business of the NMC's predecessor body the UKCC since the mid-1980s. The UKCC's Post-registration Education and Practice Project, which reported in 1994, identified two levels of practice beyond the point of registration: advanced and specialist. Explicit standards in the form of learning outcomes were set for specialist practice and a conceptual descriptor of advanced practice was offered. Rapid changes in healthcare practice, the advent of new clinical roles with titles such as nurse practitioner and advanced practitioner, the increasing number of practitioners working in very different ways and with greatly enhanced levels of responsibility in practice, and the move of post-registration education into higher education led the Council to re-examine its post-registration framework in 1996. Following a series of projects which examined the concepts of advanced and specialist practice, the Council agreed that work should be taken forward to enable it to determine and regulate a higher level of clinical practice. This work aimed to enhance the existing regulatory framework for nurses, midwives and health visitors by providing a mechanism by which users and employers could confirm whether a practitioner who claims to be able to practise at a higher level has in fact demonstrated their ability to do so.

The UKCC's standard and assessment system for the regulation of a higher level of practice in nursing, midwifery and health visiting drew upon a range of sources of data and expertise in its development. These included users, representatives from the health and social care professions, employers, research findings, and the experience of regulators in Canada, the USA, New Zealand and Australia. A process of consensus-forming was then used to develop a draft descriptor, standard and assessment system and this draft was then tested with users, the three professions and key stakeholders through a series of communication and consultation events across the four countries of the UK. This resulted in the development of a standard which identified the specific outcomes against which practitioners could be assessed, and the design of a robust assessment system. The standard and assessment system and the process of its development have been well received by the professions, employers, users and other health and social care professions as a model of good practice. City & Guilds *Affinity* was commissioned to pilot the standard and assessment system on the UKCC's behalf.

The competence-based approach the UKCC developed does not assess hours of education undertaken or subjects completed. Rather it outlines the standard expected and requires practitioners to supply evidence to demonstrate that they have achieved the standard. The focus is on the practitioner's practice rather than the process by which they acquired this ability in practice. The standard and assessment process are not tied to any particular educational programme or course. The focus of assessment is what the individual has achieved in practice, presented as evidence against the standard. The assessment is criterion-referenced, i.e. the evidence which the practitioner presents is judged against the criteria in the pilot standard. The practitioner is not judged in relation to other practitioners or in relation to their own development. The standard is set out under seven broad practice headings with criteria related to each of the headings (Table 4.3). The principles adopted by the UKCC in the specification of the assessment process included:

- A focus on achievement in practice
- A criterion-referenced model of assessment in which decisions are based on evidence from a number of sources
- The responsibility for collecting and structuring evidence to be in the hands of the practitioner seeking recognition
- A three-year re-registration cycle based on a personal development plan
- Recognition that a variety of learning opportunities will be required to support the development of competence but that there would be no prescribed education and training routes (UKCC 2002).

The pilot demonstrated that it was possible to articulate a higher level of practice in the form of a threshold and generic standard which was applicable to nursing, midwifery and health visiting, all healthcare settings and which described a level of practice not speciality or role. The assessment system enables valid and reliable assessment of individual practitioners. The pilot showed that the system was inclusive and that practitioners were able to use educational qualifications as part of their individual portfolio of evidence. The attachment of the pilot standard to the four countries' guidance on the appointment of nurse, midwife and health visitor consultant posts (see, for example, NHS Management Executive 1999) and the interest expressed by regulators from countries including Australia, New Zealand and Canada demonstrates that the leadership provided by the UKCC in this area has been recognised.

Table 4.3 Higher-level practice: practice areas and examples of criteria (UKCC 2002).

Practice headings	Criteria Practitioners working at a higher level:

(1) Providing effective healthcare	(1) Communicate effectively with individuals and groups and empower them to make informed choices about their health and healthcare
	(2) In partnership with individuals, groups and other professionals, make sound and ethical decisions balancing the interests of individuals, groups and communities
	(3) Assess individuals holistically using a range of assessment methods that are:
	  • appropriate to individuals' needs, context and culture
	  • based on research evidence and best practice

(2) Leading and developing practice	(1) Work collaboratively and in partnership with other practitioners (2) Offer appropriate advice to their own and other professions on practice, service delivery and service development (3) Support the development of knowledge and practice in their own and other professions, proactively and on request
(3) Improving quality and health outcomes	(1) Gather and interpret information from different sources and make informed judgements about its quality and appropriateness (2) Effectively synthesise knowledge and expertise related to an area of practice (3) Seize opportunities to apply new knowledge to their own and others' practice in structured ways that are capable of evaluation

(4) Innovation and changing practice	(1) Manage and facilitate change in ways that:
	  • are effective for the context and culture
	  • are consistent with standards of good practice in the UK and internationally
	  • improve practice and health outcomes
	(2) Develop appropriate strategies to make best use of resources and technology in the interests of individuals, groups and communities and to improve health outcomes
	(3) Contribute to the development of their own area of practice outside their own setting through disseminating their work to improve the health and well-being of individuals, groups and communities

Contd.

Table 4.3 *Contd.*

Practice headings	Criteria Practitioners working at a higher level:
(5) Evaluation and research	(1) Continually evaluate their own and others' practice using a range of approaches that are valid and appropriate to needs and context (2) Critically appraise and synthesise the outcomes of relevant research and evaluations and apply them to improve practice (3) Alert appropriate agencies and people to gaps in evidence and/or practice knowledge that require resolution through research
(6) Developing self and others	(1) Are proactive in developing and improving their own competence in structured ways, including reviewing practice with colleagues from other professions (2) Develop and use appropriate strategies and opportunities to share knowledge with, and influence the practice of: • colleagues in their own profession at different stages of development • practitioners from other health and social care professions whilst remaining self-aware and understanding the limits of their own competence (3) Work collaboratively with others to plan and deliver interventions to meet the learning and development needs of their own and other professions
(7) Working across professional and organisational boundaries	(1) Develop and sustain appropriate relationships, partnerships and networks to influence and improve health outcomes and healthcare delivery (2) Draw upon an appropriate range of multi-agency and interprofessional resources in their work and proactively develop new partnerships (3) Acquire new knowledge and skills and apply them in practice to provide continuity of healthcare for individuals, groups and communities, both within and across recognised professional and service boundaries

However, owing to the Council itself undergoing a period of change, regulating a higher level of practice has slipped down the agenda as the new NMC establishes itself. When and if the subject will re-emerge as a regulatory issue will depend on the new Council coping with the influx of registrations from overseas nurses to meet the shortfalls in NHS staffing and possibly the continuance of developments across the healthcare professions in anticipation of the arrival of the UK Council of Regulators. The arrival of the NMC has heralded a shift in the regulation of nursing from one largely focused on conduct to regulation that also includes continuing competence (HM Government 2002). This would bring the new Council back to the reason for developing the higher-level practice standard and associated assessment process.

A multi-professional perspective

There are a number of competence developments led by others that are multi-professional/health-sector-wide in character and might also impact on advanced nursing practice. Two examples of such developments are given below.

The sector skills council for health – Skills for Health

Skills for Health was previously the national training organisation Healthwork UK. It is in the process of developing national occupational standards/competences for a wide range of areas. These either directly include nursing, and specifically advanced nursing practice, or are likely to have an impact on it. These national occupational standards and related learning programmes and awards take a sector- and service-wide view rather than a uni-professional or nursing, view. For example, Skills for Health is developing:

- Competences for the Department of Health in England's care groups linked to the National Service Frameworks. This includes such areas as long-term care, long-term conditions, such as diabetes and renal, children's services, and services for older people
- National occupational standards for mental health that will be applicable across the UK and are intended to cover all practitioners who work in this area from any professional background and including those in health and social care
- National occupational standards for public health for both specialist practitioners where there is a need for comparability across medical and non-medical professions and for public health practice more generally. This will assist with access and progression and ensure there are sufficient individuals to meet the new public health agenda
- National occupational standards for a new breed of worker to meet the requirements of government for improving mammography screening services.

The first three examples would, by their nature, include advanced nursing practice as one of the professional groups within the ambit of the competence developments.

Agenda for Change

The Agenda for Change initiative (DoH 2000), which has been responsible for spawning the development of many local competences following the publication of the nursing-specific framework *Making a Difference* (DoH 1999), is, at the time of writing, if management and staff-side negotiations are completed successfully, soon to enter its early implementation phase. A Knowledge and Skills Framework (KSF) is in the process of development to support the consistent application of standards for all jobs in the NHS (DoH 2002). The KSF is designed to have strong links with a number of other competence-based initiatives and is seen to be important in developing a workforce focused on delivering patient-centred care and service improvements. The KSF does not seek to replicate existing work such as that on National Occupational

Standards but rather to provide a common framework which unites existing initiatives in a way that supports consistent development and appraisal of staff as they move around the service. The aim of the KSF is to produce a common way of describing applied knowledge and skills that could be used for any post in the NHS, and which gives employers and staff a common currency for use in recruitment and development.

The KSF has a number of dimensions. Some, such as communication, are expected to be relevant to all NHS jobs. These are termed 'core dimensions'. Other dimensions such as research and evaluation will apply to some jobs but not others and are known as 'specific dimensions'. Each dimension has 'level descriptors' with indicators and examples of their application attached to them. These describe the generally recognised steps in extending and applying knowledge and skills in an NHS environment. In the more detailed document, the level descriptors will be further supported by a number of criteria. References to other UK/national quality assured competences are also given.

The purpose of the KSF is to support career progression in the NHS, and subject to negotiations, possibly also pay progression. Individual staff members and their managers will be supported in their use of the KSF through a development review process which includes ongoing review of the individual applying their knowledge and skills to meet the demands of their post, followed by personal development planning, learning and development, and evaluation of that learning. It is not yet possible to assess its precise impact on the NHS in general or nursing in particular. However, from other trends in healthcare, and the interest of the current government in healthcare professionals becoming more flexible in the work they undertake, with similar flexibility in education and training to support that work, the question arises as to the extent to which competence will be used to distinguish professions or to show what they have in common.

Conclusion

This review has outlined a range of competence development initiatives being undertaken both within and outside the nursing profession. The boundaries between the health professions are becoming progressively more blurred as a result of practice and service development and government initiatives to increase the flexibility of the healthcare workforce. The UK government has become increasingly interested in competence as a means of enabling individuals to change professions and routes within professions and as a means of supporting pay and reward systems. In addition, clinical governance and a raft of other policy developments are placing a greater legal obligation on employers to ensure that their employees are fit for purpose, competent to carry out the tasks or activities they are undertaking. Consumer groups are taking a much more active interest in how healthcare is provided and in the competence of individual practitioners delivering services, all of which suggest the need for further national development of robust performance outcome models of competence to assess advanced practice which may need to be multi-professional rather than uni-disciplinary in nature. The following questions invite you to continue to consider the issues that we have raised here.

? **Key questions for Chapter 4**

In your field of practice:

(1) What types of competence are most useful to advanced practitioners and how might these be assessed?
(2) In what ways could the advantages and disadvantages of uni-professional and multi-professional approaches to competence, in the development of advanced practice, be determined?
(3) What strategies could advanced practitioners use to influence the setting of standards and competences by agencies outside nursing?

References

Bloom, B.S. (ed.) (1956) *Taxonomy of Educational Objectives: The Classification of Educational Goals. Handbook I: Cognitive Domain.* New York: Longmans, Green.

Boak, G. (1998) Benchmarks for competency models. *Competency*, 5 (2). London: IRS.

DoH (1999) *Making a Difference: Strengthening the Nursing, Midwifery and Health Visiting Contribution to Health and Healthcare.* London: DoH.

DoH (2000) *Agenda for Change: Modernising the NHS Pay System. Joint Framework of Principles and Agreed Statement on the Way Forward.* London: DoH.

DoH (2002) *Agenda for Change: Knowledge and Skills Framework*, Note to the Service, March.

HM Government (2002) The Nursing and Midwifery Order 2001, No. 253. London: The Stationery Office.

Management Charter Initiative (1997) *Management Standards*, Manage People Key Role C, p. 187. Kent.

Mitchell, L. (2000) Paper presented to the UKCC's HLP Steering Group, UKCC. Unpublished.

NHS Management Executive (1999) *Nurse, Midwife and Health Visitor Consultants: Establishing Posts and Making Appointments*, Health Service Circular 1999/217. Leeds: NHS Executive.

NONPF (1995) *Advanced Nursing Practice: Curriculum Guidelines and Program Standards for Nurse Practitioner Education.* Washington, DC: NONPF.

RCN (2000) *Information Pack on the Expert Practice Project and Pilot.* London: RCN.

RCN (2002) *Nurse Practitioners: An RCN Guide to the Nurse Practitioner Role, Competencies and Programme Accreditation.* London: RCN.

UKCC (1999) *Fitness for Practice: The UKCC Commission for Nursing and Midwifery Education.* London: UKCC.

UKCC (2002) *Report of the Higher Level of Practice Pilot and Project.* London: UKCC.

Chapter 5

Clinical Practice Benchmarking and Advanced Practice

Sarah Coleman and Jane Fox

Introduction

The dimension of leadership within advanced practice requires the practitioner to engage in critical analysis of patient care and outcomes. Such analysis provides the advanced practitioner with the information required both to challenge the status quo and to work effectively within the organisation. One of the strategies through which critical analysis can be undertaken is clinical benchmarking. This chapter introduces the role of the advanced practitioner in the context of clinical benchmarking, together with a review of the developmental forces and environment for this initiative. Clinical benchmarking can be defined as 'a quality initiative that seeks to learn from others' best practice' (Cole *et al.* 2000). This is not a new concept but has been used for many years to compare and monitor performance and standards in industry. One editorial describes it as 'a euphemism for legally ripping off someone else's idea, then improving on it' (Port & Smith 1992).

Attempts to quantify the *quality* of essential nursing care have been made using clinical audit against set standards. This approach to monitoring of care quality does not explore the qualitative perspective. Recent government initiatives have led to emphasis on the importance of getting the basics right. The quality of care has received increasing attention through complaints upheld by the ombudsman. The aim of clinical benchmarking is 'to help improve . . . the quality of fundamental and essential aspects of care' (DoH 2001).

Context and influential forces

Inevitably, the role of the advanced and specialist nursing practitioner and specifically the use of clinical benchmarking within this are subject to influence by a number of forces. This section of the chapter seeks to consider the nature and interrelationship of such forces. Recognition that nursing roles are subject to influence by diverse forces, both external and internal to the profession, is not new, although arguably, entry into a new millennium gave particular emphasis to such deliberations, this being characterised by, for example, Henderson (2001: 722) who suggested that globalisation in the twenty-first century marked a new era of challenge for nursing:

> The new era is characterised by worldwide changes of a magnitude never seen before, mostly in the form of expanding world markets, instantaneous communication, travel at the speed of sound, political realignments, changing demographics and technological transformations.

If such a position is accepted then, clearly, the individual forces for change are diverse and to some extent interdependent, forming a complex tapestry within which nursing, and specifically specialist/advanced practice, takes place. It is therefore beyond the scope of this chapter to explore each force for change to any great extent; all that can be attempted is an overview. To this end it is perhaps helpful to characterise such forces as being either societal, NHS organisational, or professional in nature, although such categories are not seen as mutually exclusive. Table 5.1 summarises significant influential forces which are considered in more depth below.

Societal forces

Societal change since the 1960s has seen advancement in information access through greater availability of telecommunication, information highways, ease of travel and multinational agencies/organisations, resulting in a related increased demand by the public for information regarding the quality and delivery of all public services, including that of healthcare. Such a demand has resulted in a greater range and amount of published and comparative information, for example in the form of annual reports, league tables and web pages dedicated to public services. A climate of greater transparency has been generated by which public expenditure upon health and other public services is questioned particularly in the context of efficiency, quality and appropriateness to changing need. This transparency, modernisation of the delivery of public services and its underpinning culture has emerged as a central tenet of policy in relation to many public services, such a transformation in the context of healthcare having its origins in the ideologies of the NHS as first envisaged, the quasi-market of the 1980s and 1990s, and the current health citizenship or third way of Labour government's policy (Antrobus 1997; Ranade 1997; Ham 1999; Hogg 1999; Giddens

Table 5.1 Influential forces for change.

Societal	NHS organisational	Professional
• Impact of globalisation	• Central *vis-à-vis* devolved authority	
• Reforms and modernisation of all public services	• Changing NHS policy and values	• Review and reinforcement of professional regulation
• Societal diversity	• Modernisation agenda	• Evidencing role/ interdisciplinary boundaries, e.g. nurse consultants, advanced practitioners
• Increased public demand for access to information	• Skill and workforce changes/diversity	• Partnership with patients and clients in care delivery
• Media attention to perceived healthcare failures: threat to public confidence	• Clinical governance and risk management	• Review of professional knowledge and identity
• Public sector expenditure agendas	• IM&T (information management and technology) increased capability	• Increased attention to clinical and professional leadership capabilities
• Changes to quality assurance monitoring arrangements in other public sectors, e.g. education	• Increased emphasis upon evidence as a basis for delivery of care (CHIE, NICE)	• Evidence-based practice
	• Acceptance/wider use of audit	
	• Increased attention to value for money	

2000). Accordingly, changes in both ideology and the delivery of public services, including health, are subject to increasing public debate and media attention. Commonly such debates centre upon questions of state/individual/private sector contribution to services, prioritisation of services in the context of resource constraints, and, above all, quality assurance and public safety/satisfaction in relation to these. The emergence of quality as a pivotal societal agenda in relation to public services, including health, is perhaps inevitable, resulting in the NHS seeking strategies to secure quality and thereby public confidence.

NHS organisational forces

If the claim for the centrality of quality on the public agenda is accepted then the rationale for particular changes within the NHS at large becomes evident. The search for quality assurance and enhancement in the NHS is potentially subject to tension created by the desire both to secure a genuinely national service which meets the needs of citizens in an equitable and common way and to be sufficiently responsive to different needs and historical legacies locally. Thus a tension between centralised and decentralised structures and quality arrangements exists, this tension being envisaged in the early 1990s by authors such as Bartlet *et al.* (1994), Pollit *et al.* (1998) and Spires (1995). Such authors acknowledged that in order to be assured of national standards within a decentralised service, increasingly sophisticated and wide-ranging central devices for measuring local quality against national norms would be developed. They suggested that such regulatory devices could include clinical guidelines, peer accreditation, national published service standards, and self-governance require-ments. As Pollit *et al.* (1998: 163) argue: 'the decentralisation was accompanied by significant measures of centralisation'.

More recently, the expansion, utility and relevance of such developed quality measures and tables to the public and specifically the health professional and patient in isolation as a basis for informing health decisions has been questioned (Anthony 2000) and subject to further enquiry. Examples of this include Attree's (2001) exploration of quality criteria used by health professionals, managers and patients, and Turrill's (2000) review of whether standardised neonatal care is possible. Additionally, such questioning is exemplified by Bell (2001: 171) who suggests that, 'as citizens and individuals there is little we can do with information about how well the NHS is doing'. Such a view may in part explain why the NHS has sought to place quality measures in the context of clinical governance rather than view them as isolated quality assurance strategies, because 'it is no longer satisfactory for developments to exist in a vacuum or indeed for individuals to act in a vacuum' (Scott 2001: 58). Indeed, the central relationship of both internal and external mechanisms for improving quality within clinical governance has been widely acknowledged, Walshe (1998), Swage (2000), and Lugon and Secker-Walker (1999) being examples of authors who adopt this view.

Arguably, a further force for the development of quality tests and measures which can be applied to different care situations is the change and diversity of the NHS workforce and skill mix contained within this. Such changes imply that there can be considerable local diversity in the care team delivering direct patient care in respect of healthcare support workers *vis-à-vis* registered nurses, other healthcare professionals, and level of educational/professional knowledge and skill. Such changes are forecast to increase in the context of common education programmes for professionals, with a predicted retirement rate of approximately 25% among registered nurses over the five years to 2007 (Akid 2002). Clearly, the emergence of the specialist and advanced practitioner role is one example of wider workforce change within the NHS, albeit a significant one, particularly if Castledine's (2002) suggestion that coordinating and organising the healthcare team is one of seven major aspects of the role.

A further force of change within the NHS as a whole and one worthy of highlighting is the increased emphasis upon evidence as a basis for care. This is manifested in organisational studies with specific terms of reference relating to evidence, notably those of the National Institute for Clinical Excellence (NICE). Scott (2001: 45) states that, 'the NICE has been established to set standards by developing clinical guidelines based on evidence of clinical and cost effectiveness to agree associated audit methodologies from good practice'. Reciprocally, as identified above, audit of the clinical environment and practice is now accepted and is embedded in the quality assurance approach of the NHS as a whole (Kogan *et al.* 1995).

Professional forces

Both societal and NHS organisational forces impact upon the profession as a whole, influencing professional values, knowledge and accepted working practices, reflecting Johnston's (1999) view that nursing in England today has the wind of change behind it. Certainly, it can be claimed that in the context of considerable societal and organisational change there has been extensive professional debate and discourse within nursing and midwifery. These debates have embraced such issues as the profession's identity (Tschudin 1999), philosophical position and values (Edwards 1998), educational requirements (Birchenall 2002; Wharrad *et al.* 2002), and professional regulation (Munroe 2002). Additionally, an emerging pivotal issue of professional concern is the relationship between the role of evidence-based practice, particularly in the context of changing/extended role, the challenge of implementing research funding in practice and the professional leadership required to facilitate the use of evidence-based practice (Bowles & Bowles 2000; Mahoney 2001; Thompson *et al.* 2001; French 2002; Rolfe 2002). Arguably the underlying issue to such debates is the quest for appropriate professional standards and approaches to ensure the quality of care delivered in the face of ever increasing professional and care diversity. It is therefore in this context that clinical benchmarking takes centre stage as a professional issue and more specifically has relevance to specialist and advanced practice.

The benchmarking cycle

The benchmark against which practice is compared is the 'best practice' achievable, defined by consensus opinion. This may include evidence from research studies, expert opinion or clinical experience. Levels of evidence are graded A–C or D (Phillips *et al.* 2001).

Eight areas of care were approached in the initial document from the Department of Health (DoH 2001). These were:

- Principles of self-care
- Food and nutrition
- Personal and oral hygiene
- Continence and bladder and bowel care
- Pressure ulcers
- Record-keeping
- Safety of clients/patients with mental health needs in acute mental health and general hospital settings
- Privacy and dignity

The benchmarking cycle is composed of a series of steps (Fig. 5.1). Areas of practice to be explored are agreed. A multidisciplinary team is established with commitment

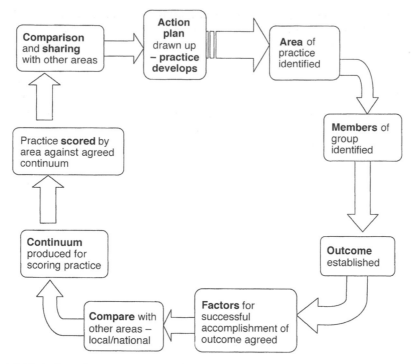

Fig. 5.1   The benchmarking cycle (adapted from DoH 2001).

for regular meetings. The outcome is decided and factors which contribute to the completion of the outcome are identified. Evidence is collected from a selection of clinical areas, regional and national examples, and a continuum is established to score individual areas' practices. Comparison of actual practice with the continuum then takes place, with scores being awarded. This information is then shared locally and action plans for improvements and practice development are agreed. These are then disseminated.

Advanced practitioner role

The role of the advanced nurse practitioner (ANP) as identified by McGee and Castledine (1999) contains key elements of clinical practice, teaching, research, advising and management. The differences seen between the role of the ANP and the specialist nurse lay mainly in the approach to the clinical practice elements of the role. ANPs perform advanced assessments, make referrals, conduct nurse-led clinics, order investigations, prescribe and treat patients, whereas specialist nurses are more involved with performing the specialist care associated with diagnosing and treating patients' problems and with providing direct care.

Identifying best practice

In the clinical setting where benchmarking activity is in progress, the ANPs skills are vital in contributing to identifying best practice, acting as a resource and consultant[1] in their specialist field, and implementing change based on evidence-based findings. Dissemination of best practice at conferences and other forums facilitate improvements in quality of nursing care. This method of benchmarking has been evident in an informal way in specialist/advanced practice for several years. Clinical benchmarking provides the framework to evaluate the qualitative aspects of the care we deliver – enabling us to strive for excellence by comparison and sharing with others. In identifying best practice, all levels of evidence must be considered (Ellis 2000a). This is particularly pertinent when there is no research base to support procedures or processes used, but reliance is placed on past practice and outcomes.

Networking and compiling action plans

Sharing data obtained through benchmarking practice in an open manner ensures that continual quality improvement occurs, as has been demonstrated in paediatric care in the north-west of England (Ellis 2000a). The leadership qualities of the ANP are then instrumental in encouraging the multidisciplinary team to work together to implement the best practices identified. Teaching and communicating evidence-based practice is an inherent part of the ANPs role. Such nurses are actively engaged in education of all grades of nursing and medical staff, and this puts them in a pivotal position for the successful dissemination and uptake of evidence-based practice within the specialist setting (Fig. 5.2). One method advocated for dissemination is that of using link nurses in clinical areas (Ellis 2000b), an approach frequently used in practice such as infection control. Networking across traditional boundaries between disciplines, education and trusts facilitates clinical supervision, reduces the potential theory/practice divide whilst enabling the practice of benchmarking to take place, and can provide a supportive network in itself (Sawley & Hale 1998).

Role development and contribution to clinical benchmarking

There is a lack of published material relating to the contribution of ANPs in the benchmarking process. Anecdotal evidence suggests that there is a lack of direct involvement of ANPs with the benchmarking process, although they may see the framework as an excellent method for continuous improvement of nursing care. This is exemplified by the comments of one ANP working in the context of wound care:

> Clinical benchmarking begins to challenge and legitimises the fundamentals of nursing practice. It does this by questioning our application of evidence-based healthcare 'what we know' and 'what we do' in an area that has sometimes been considered as basic nursing care. As an advanced practitioner I see this as a unique opportunity to explore the issue of quality within nursing and in relation to my role, the whole issue of pressure ulcer damage and prevention. There has been an assumption that this area of care is good and has been 'taken

---

[1] There is a growing distinction between the role of the ANP as consultant and the future of the role of 'nurse consultant'.

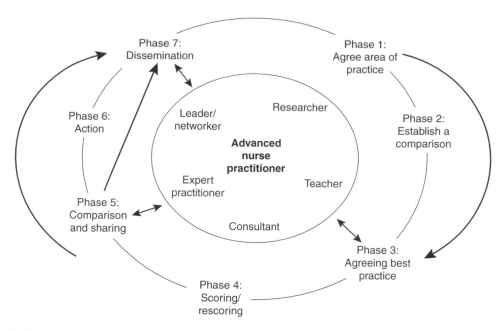

Fig. 5.2   Relationship between the clinical benchmarking cycle and the advanced nurse practitioner role.

for granted' with the prevention of pressure ulcers being viewed as something to be delegated. This is a real opportunity through leadership to create the culture. The culture of openness, sharing, reflecting, challenging constructively, learning and of really moving practice forward.
(Jackie Steven-Haynes, Lecturer/Practitioner in Tissue Viability, Worcestershire Primary Care Trust (2002))

Trusts have identified some of the advantages of employing ANPs as: improving patient care, increasing creativity in care provision and pioneering new ideas (McGee & Castledine 1999). These activities are seen to be fundamental concepts to clinical benchmarking processes. It is appropriate therefore to question why there appears to be a reluctance to involve ANPs in clinical benchmarking.

Woods (1999) describes a longitudinal study over two years exploring the ANPs development, the findings of which showed that ANPs passed through three stages in their transition from experienced nurse to advanced nurse practitioner. These were:

- Stage 1: *the idealism of reconstruction*. At this stage the ANPs had high expectations of the role, different people in the organisation had different expectations of the role, and stakeholders lacked clarity in the role objectives, scope of practice and individual responsibilities and anticipated outcomes of practice. This led to inter- and intraprofessional conflict and frustration: there were competing institutional and personal agendas.
- Stage 2: *organisational governance*. This occurred in the first year of the role and was defined as 'reality shock'. Initial expectations had not been met, goals and para-

meters of the role were negotiated with managerial and medical staff, and individuals felt controlled by dominant stakeholders. The organisational agenda and availability of resources limited the extent of role transition.

- Stage 3: *resolution*. This occurred in the second year of the role and was characterised by acceptance and implementation. The ANPs acknowledge the limitations of the role imposed through organisational governance. Other stakeholders accept the ANPs in performance of their role. ANPs are seen to be most effective at this stage. The ANP then becomes a key stakeholder and begins to renegotiate the parameters of their role with the other stakeholders.

If this model of development of ANPs is correct then perhaps ANPs are unable to contribute to the benchmarking process in an autonomous way until they reach the 'resolution' stage (stage 3) of role development. With many ANPs still new in post, and with the introduction of nurse consultants, many are still in the stage of 'organisational governance' (stage 2). The ability of ANPs in this stage to take an effective role in benchmarking is therefore limited. From their perspective, other aspects of the role, such as running clinics and prescribing and carrying out treatments traditionally carried out by junior doctors, take precedence. With continual processes of change, reorganisation and political directives, the clinical arena appears to be in a state of constant flux with roles continually being challenged. A recent review by the Kings Fund found that the past five years of government health policy was: 'an overwhelming impression of relentless, almost hyperactive intervention' (Appleby & Coote 2002).

Perhaps this situation limits full implementation and evaluation of initiatives; accordingly, unless identified as a managerial priority, clinical benchmarking appears to be taking a back seat in the queue for implementation. Successful implementation of clinical benchmarking has been shown to be dependent on practitioner commitment and managerial support (Ellis 2000b). Again, anecdotal evidence suggests that many ANPs may see the eight areas identified in 'essence of care' (DoH 2001) as too generalist to warrant their involvement. They have other priorities. Evidence from the north of England suggests that staff were 'extremely hesitant about the value of benchmarking as nothing appeared to be happening' (Ellis 2000b). This may be the opinion of ANPs not involved in their trust's current initiatives.

Future development of benchmarking within the ANP role

The future of the ANP role is further discussed in Chapter 18. Castledine (1998) warned of the dangers of nurse specialists focusing their work 'too much on the medical model and the technical procedures associated with that approach'. He foresaw the fact that essential nursing care was being neglected. He went on to say: 'nurse specialists of the future should be acting as clinical leaders, promoting the development and application of the essentials of nursing'. This is where the role of the ANP lies within the context of clinical benchmarking (Fig. 5.2). Manley (2000) builds on these key elements of practice described earlier by Castledine in her description of the nurse consultant role as an expert practitioner; an educator and enabler of others; a researcher, expert and process consultant; and transformational leader. She further describes three core outcomes: a transformational culture (where change becomes a way of life), empowered staff, and practice development. These three areas reflect the key requirements for successful implementation of clinical benchmarking. It is imperative, therefore, that advanced practitioners and nurse consultants take on the challenge of the *Essence of Care* (DoH 2001) document at a strategic level.

Conclusion

As benchmarking spreads to involve more specialist areas of practice such as wound care, specialist and advanced practitioners by default become involved. As role models and advocates of best practice, ANPs must become engaged in the formal processes of clinical benchmarking. However, if they do not involve themselves in the process of some of the more fundamental areas of nursing care being approached initially, such as privacy and dignity, nutrition and documentation, they will not understand the process in sufficient depth to address more specialist areas of practice within their remit. If they continue to ignore benchmarking within their roles, they are conspiring to ignore basic nursing care issues and belying its importance. This is a disservice to the patient and the nursing profession. We hope that the following questions will help practitioners to further consider their role in benchmarking.

 Key questions for Chapter 5

In your field of practice:

(1) What are the opportunities open to advanced practitioners to become involved in clinical benchmarking?
(2) In what ways do you think advanced practitioners could contribute to clinical practice benchmarking in essential and specialist nursing care?
(3) How might the advanced practitioner facilitate an evidence-based culture for practice?

References

Akid, M. (2002) Number of student nurses needs to double. *Nursing Times*, 98(11): 7.
Anthony, D. (2000) Clinical guidelines: an increase in interest in the UK. *Clinical Effectiveness in Nursing*, 4: 198–204.
Antrobus, S. (1997) An analysis of nursing in context: the effects of current health policy. *Journal of Advanced Nursing*, 25(3): 447–53.
Appleby, J. & Coote, A. (2002) *Five-year Health Check: A Review of Health Policy, 1997–2002*. London: Kings Fund.
Attree, M. (2001) A study of the criteria used by healthcare professionals, managers and patients to represent and evaluate quality care. *Journal of Nursing Management* 9, 67–78.

Bartlett, W., Propper, C., Wilson, D. & Grand, L. (1994) *Quasi Markets in the Welfare State*. Bristol: SAUS Publications.

Bell, A. (2001) Measure for measure, or how we can judge the NHS. *British Journal of Health Care Management*, 6(4) 170–71.

Birchenhall, P. (2002) Editorial. Diversity a driving force in curriculum development. *Nurse Education Today*, 22(1): 1–2.

Bowles, A. & Bowles, N.B. (2000) A comparative study of transformational leadership in nursing development units and conventional clinical settings. *Journal of Nursing Management*, 8(2): 69–76.

Castledine, G. (1998) The future of specialist and advanced practice. In: *Advanced and Specialist Nursing Practice* (eds G. Castledine & P. McGee), pp. 225–32. Oxford: Blackwell Science.

Castledine, G. (2002) The important aspects of nurse specialist roles. *British Journal of Nursing*, 11(5): 350.

Cole, N., Tucker, L.J. & Foxcroft, D. (2000) Benchmarking evidence-based nursing. *NT Research* 5(5): 336–45.

DoH (2001) *The Essence of Care: Patient-focused Benchmarking for Health Care Practitioners*. London: DoH.

Edwards, S.D. (1998) *Philosophical Issues in Nursing*. Basingstoke: Macmillan.

Ellis, J. (2000a) Sharing the evidence: clinical practice benchmarking to improve continuously the quality of care. *Journal of Advanced Nursing*, 32(1): 215–25.

Ellis, J. (2000b) Making a difference to practice: clinical benchmarking. Part 2. *Nursing Standard*, 14(33): 32–5.

French, P. (2002) What is the evidence on evidence-based nursing? An epistemological concern. *Journal of Advanced Nursing*, 37(3): 250–57.

Giddens, A. (2000) *The Third Way and Its Critics*. Cambridge: Polity Press.

Ham, C. (1999) *Health Policy in Britain: Public Policy and Politics*, 4th edn. Basingstoke: Macmillan.

Henderson, V. (2001) Oration. Nursing: A new era for action. *Journal of Advanced Nursing*, 36(6): 722–76.

Hogg, C. (1999) *Patients, Power and Politics: from patients to citizens*. London: Sage.

Johnston, C. (1999) Board Editorial. *Nursing Times Research*, 4(1): 404.

Kogan, M., Redfern, S., Kober, A., Norman, I., Packwood, T. & Robinson, S. (1995) *Making Use of Clinical Audit*. Buckingham: Open University Press.

Lugon, M.& Secker-Walker, J. (eds) (1999) *Clinical Governance: Making It Happen*. London: RSM Press.

Mahoney, J. (2001) Leadership skills for the 21st century. *Journal of Nursing Management*, 9(5): 269–71.

Manley, K. (2000) Organisational culture and consultant nurse outcomes. Part 1: Organisational culture. *Nursing Standard*, 14(36): 34–8.

McGee, P. & Castledine, G. (1999) A survey of specialist and advanced nursing practice in the UK. *British Journal of Nursing*, 8(16): 1074–8.

Munroe, R. (2002) Have you got the perfect body? *Nursing Times*, 98(11): 14.

Phillips, B., Ball, C., Sackett, D. et al. (2001) *Levels of Evidence and Grades of Recommendations*. Oxford: Centre for Evidence-based Medicine. Available at http://www.cebm.net/levels of evidence.asp

Pollitt, C., Birchall, J. & Putman, K. (1998) *Decentralising Public Service Management*. Basingstoke: Macmillan.

Port, O. & G. Smith (1992) Beg, borrow ... and benchmark. *Business Week*, 30 November.

Ranade, W. (1997) *A Future for the NHS? Health Care for the Millennium*, 2nd edn. Harlow: Longman.

Rolfe, G. (2002) Faking a difference: evidence-based nursing and the illusion of diversity. *Nurse Education Today*, 22(1): 3–12.

Sawley, L. & Hale, K. (1998) Effective group support: an innovative network in Lancashire. *Journal of Child Health Care*, 2(3): 187–9.

Scott, I. (2001) Clinical governance: a framework and models for practice. In: *Challenges in Clinical Practice Professional Developments in Nursing* (eds V. Bishop & I. Scott), p. 45. Basingstoke: Palgrave.

Spires, J. (1995) *The Invisible Hospital and the Secret Garden: An Insider's Commentary on the NHS Reforms.* Oxford: Radcliffe Medical Press.

Swage, T. (2000) *Clinical Governance in Health Care Practice.* Oxford: Butterworth-Heinemann.

Thompson, C., McCoughan, D., Callum, N., Sheldon, T.A., Malhall, A. & Thompson, D.R. (2001) The accessibility of research-based knowledge for nurses in United Kingdom acute care setting. *Journal of Advanced Nursing*, 36(1): 11–22.

Tschudin, V. (1999) *Nursing Matters: Reclaiming Our Professional Identity.* Basingstoke: Macmillan.

Turrill, S. (2000) Is access to a standardised neonatal intensive care possible? *Journal of Nursing Management*, 8: 49–56.

Walshe, K. (1998) Clinical governance: what does it really mean? *Health Services Management Centre Newsletter*, 4(2): 1–2.

Wharrad, H., Clifford, C., Harsburgh, M., Kefefian, S. & Lee, J. (2002) Global network explores diversity and opportunity in nurse education. *Nurse Education Today*, 22(1): 15–23.

Woods, L. (1999) The contingent nature of advanced nursing practice. *Journal of Advanced Nursing*, 30(1): 121–8.

Chapter 6

Supervision and Leadership in Advanced Nursing Practice

Ann Close

Introduction

In Chapter 3 of this book, McGee and Castledine assert that two of the core elements of advanced practice are the ability to challenge professional boundaries and to pioneer innovations. Inherent in both these abilities is the concept of leadership that, in the context of modern healthcare, requires the advanced practitioner to analyse complex situations and functions, create new possibilities and to communicate these to others as both desirable and achievable. Leadership is, therefore, contingent upon a high level of interpersonal competence that enables others not only to understand what the leader intends but also to feel motivated to share in making that intention a reality. Leaders, by definition, have followers. They also, through education and experience, have the professional maturity needed to challenge the status quo and to try something new, even if this means taking a chance on something that may or may not succeed.

This chapter begins by examining theoretical ideas about leadership, and in particular, four sub-elements defined by Yates (1999) as 'the four Es': envisioning, enabling, empowering and energising. Each of these is discussed and related to contextual issues such as the organisational setting and the qualities required by the leader. Styles of leadership are then addressed with particular reference to democratic and transformational approaches that facilitate followers to actively participate as co-owners of the vision and thus to demonstrate commitment to it. In the second part of the chapter the emphasis is on the practical dimensions of leadership in healthcare, with an overview of initiatives, such as the introduction of the Leadership Centre by the NHS Modernisation Agency, which have been used in the NHS to identify potential leaders and help those individuals to develop their skills. Leadership initiatives aimed specifically at nurses, such as the Leading Empowered Organisations programme, are also discussed. The next part of the chapter addresses issues that are related to leadership. These include differentiating leadership from management, and identifying the support that leaders need if they are to achieve their aims. Finally, the chapter presents a discussion of the ways in which advanced practitioners can provide clinical and professional leadership both within their own local sphere of influence and in the national arena.

Characteristics of leadership

Yates (1999), and others such as Adair (1984), Armstrong (1994), O'Connor (1994) and Cole (1997), argue that leadership is mostly about understanding people, especially about getting them working together, and about listening and making real connections with them. It also depends on having a unique vision, making strategic choices, designing and enabling an organisation to get the job done. Yates identified 'four Es' of leadership:

- *Envisioning*: creating a vision and developing a plan to achieve it.
- *Enabling*: choosing the right people with the necessary skills to get the job done and rewarding them for it.
- *Empowering*: people to achieve the vision in a two-way contract between the leader and the followers in which successes, failures, rewards and sanctions are defined, and both are held mutually accountable.
- *Energising*: people to act by expressing the vision, often in a charismatic way, as a story that builds up understanding and motivates the followers into action.

Envisioning and energising

The vision is the essential component that provides a common purpose that inspires the team to act. Handy (1991) argues that the vision has a number of key characteristics. First, it must be new, something different. If it is merely a duplicate of the present or is a replica of what someone else is doing, it is not a vision. Second, the vision must make sense to others, capture people's imagination but still be in the bounds of possibility. Third, it must be understandable and stick in people's minds so that they remember it. Fourth, the leader must live the vision, show that they believe in it, but, finally, remember that achieving it is the work of others – followers – without whom it will remain a dream. Vision, therefore, has a practical component in terms of planning and setting goals.

Enabling and empowering

Leaders have followers. The aim of the leader is to develop a team of followers that bonds and works collaboratively and willingly towards the achievement of the vision. This can occur within a small multidisciplinary team, community, ward, department or an entire organisation. Covey (1992) describes this as achieving 'interdependence' which is characterised by a feeling of 'we can do it, we can cooperate, we can combine our talents and abilities and create something greater together'. Interdependence, therefore, is a concept that leaders should aim to create in the team, as it will accomplish far more than each member could achieve alone.

Interdependence, however, does not happen without effort and commitment, and the leader has to create positive relationships and mutual respect with and between group members. Leaders should aim to achieve a balance between the needs of individuals and the work to be done by them. This requires finding the time to listen to team members in order to begin to understand what motivates them, identifying what will make the job sufficiently challenging to give them a sense of personal achievement, what values they have and what rewards are important to them. If leaders understand the frustration, limitations and drivers of their team members then they are better able to provide the necessary support. Enabling is thus a way of breaking down barriers and addressing concerns proactively.

Team members also need to know what is expected of them, what are the objectives and standards they should work to, what is their authority for making decisions and what degree of control will be exercised over them. Communication is a key element in clarifying these issues and developing a team spirit. O'Connor (1994) identifies five features necessary for effective communication. It should be:

- Goal-directed
- Coherent – consistent, clear and logical
- Appropriate to the situation
- Controlled
- Able to be learned – coaching and paraphrasing can create understanding

Opportunities for team members to seek clarification, guidance and receive feedback are essential. One-to-one discussions, team meetings, informal chats, written information and many other kinds of interaction may achieve this. Internal and external networking is also useful in obtaining support, seeking new ideas and widening horizons.

The organisational context

Leadership is a dynamic process influenced by the situation and context in which it is taking place, by the work or tasks to be done and by the attributes of the leader (Cole

1997). Different organisations have different cultures, values and ways of working, including different leadership and management styles. There are often diverse structures, procedures, methods of reward and punishment and ways of behaving towards each other. These organisational norms can have a significant impact on what can be done and what can be achieved, and it is important that they are carefully considered by people who are in leadership positions, as they should influence how those individuals act. People need to be able to identify positively with the part of the organisation in which they work and understand how they contribute to it. This will help to generate a feeling of ownership and pride that will encourage motivation and achievement. It is important that leaders are able to exercise influence in an organisation. Rowntree (1989) identifies eight sources of power in an organisation:

- Resource power – having authority for money, staff and facilities
- Information power – having access to information that others do not have
- Position power – related to title or position in an organisation
- Proxy power – being a representative of an authority figure
- Expert power – depends on personal talents, skills and experience of the individual
- Personality power – charismatic people who inspire others
- Physical power – this is from some physical attribute such as body language that intimidates people
- Favour power – requires the paying back of past favours

Plant (1987) adds two other sources of power:

- Reward power – the power to reward financially or with promotion or recognition
- Connection power – from access to networks across the organisation and beyond

Leaders may display one or more types of power, and leaders who draw on more than one power source strengthen their position. However, there is a danger that individuals with several power sources become difficult to challenge, and leadership of the team may become problematical. Leaders may also need to seek support from other people with power. This requires them to understand the politics of the organisation and identify the key decision-makers. They need to work out who needs to be influenced, who is supportive, who is likely to put up barriers and what tactics can be used to remove these. Although all these power sources may be useful, they do not necessarily make the most of the team. Waitley (1994) argues that real power comes from empowering others. Whether it is possible to invest power in others is debatable and is perhaps an artificial argument. What is important is that leaders are able to create situations in which members of staff feel valued and there are opportunities for them to grow. Many people just want the freedom and autonomy to get on with their jobs. All they need is for the leader to set the direction of travel, the boundaries in which they have authority to operate, and to be a sounding board to discuss ideas.

Qualities of the leader

The overall aim of a leader is to perform the tasks and achieve the targets that arise from the vision. There are many qualities that have been identified as being useful in leaders:

- *Expertise.* Lock (1992) suggests that a record of success in a particular specialisation combined with a broader view of how this links with other specialities is important. This is enhanced when the individual is known and respected in the organisation.
- *Effective communication.* The key is in listening and asking questions in order to understand team members, the tasks to be done and the context or situation within the organisation. Being open-minded and honest is more likely to attract a similar response from colleagues than if a pre-judgement is made. It is important not to penalise people or to discourage them from asking questions or making suggestions.
- *Enabling others.* This requires the leader to be clear on what they are trying to achieve. It may also require the leader to help colleagues to develop skills by training, coaching, guiding and supporting them. Changing leadership style to suit a particular situation will be helpful.
- *Organisational abilities.* These include being able to manage time efficiently and being able to focus attention on the job in hand and to meet agreed deadlines within the resources allocated.
- *Personal qualities.* These include commitment, flexibility, honesty and a willingness to take calculated risks. In addition, the ability to resolve conflict, make a presentation and negotiate is helpful.
- *Self-awareness.* This is possibly one of the most important attributes. It is vital that leaders recognise that their behaviour is a product of their own conscious choices based on their values and it cannot be blamed on circumstances, conditions or conditioning. Leaders should develop self-confidence in their own ability and recognise their strengths and weaknesses but have a realistic recognition of when they have reached their limits and need help. They should also develop an awareness of how well they are able to understand other people and how much they can rely on their own judgement. In some situations, leadership is not necessarily confined to one person but may be shared (Cole 1997), and the effective leader should be able to recognise when handing over the leadership function to another is beneficial.

Styles of leadership

There is general agreement that there is no one best style of leadership because so much of leadership depends on the individual. Leaders behave in certain ways because of their personal traits. Charisma is probably one of the most notable of these traits and there are many famous and infamous charismatic leaders such as Kennedy, Churchill and Hitler who have relied on their aura, personality and inspirational qualities. These are natural characteristics but experience has shown these individuals how best to use them. Advocates of charismatic styles of leadership are more likely to seek leaders through selection processes. Some organisations, including the NHS, use personality and psychomotor testing as indicators of whether a prospective employee has the required leadership attributes.

Contingency approaches to leadership are based on the philosophy that leaders adapt their individual styles to meet the needs of the situation.

- *Democratic leaders* tend to be more people-orientated and encourage participation and freedom of expression by all members of the team. They involve themselves in decision-making and rely on their know-how and persuasive ability rather than their position. They are supportive to the team's efforts in accomplishing goals by helping, guiding and coaching team members. Although this style is likely to be more effective in creating group cohesion and productivity, it can alienate 'action-oriented' people because discussion takes time and slows progress.
- *Autocratic leaders* focus on getting the task done on time and within budget, and their concern for people tends to be secondary. They are directing and give precise instructions and provide a tight, disciplined environment that allows no scope for initiative. On occasions, such as in an emergency or when team members have little experience, teams can benefit from being told what to do. This style, however, is uncomfortable for people who want to contribute ideas and information.
- *Laissez-faire or permissive leaders* hand over the responsibility for decision-making and problem-solving to the team. This style is useful when working with an experienced team who respond well to a structure-free environment.
- *Transactional leaders* function in an ordered and predictable environment. They agree goals with team members and reward them in a way that matches their achievement. They tend only to react when problems occur which means feedback is usually negative rather than positive.
- *Transformational leaders* use motivation to encourage others to strive for higher goals and standards. They are able to share their vision with staff in a language that they understand and in a way that appeals to their values and beliefs. They stimulate team members by questioning and challenging them and so develop in them a willingness to participate and commitment to achieving the goals.

Effective leadership requires flexibility and an ability to move between the leadership styles using a combination of one or more approaches. Success depends on the situation and the leader's ability to understand it and act accordingly.

Leadership development in healthcare

The NHS has encouraged the development of leadership through a wide range of programmes, many of which have been aimed at nurses. There are a number of common themes in these programmes:

- *Focus on self-awareness.* A variety of tools are used to encourage participants to understand how and why they react and behave in a certain way with a view to helping them manage themselves more effectively. These tools include:

- ○ personality tests such as Myers Briggs type indicators (Briggs & Briggs Myers 1976)
- ○ 360 degree feedback where colleagues, including peers, subordinates and seniors who work with the individual inside or outside the organisation, are asked for their views on various aspects of the individual's way of working
- ○ questionnaires to identify learning and leadership styles
- *Personal development planning* is used to build on strengths and help the individual overcome or lessen weaknesses.
- *Political awareness.* This is essential to leaders who must understand the relationship between central government, the Department of Health, strategic health authorities, primary care trusts and other trusts. Leaders should understand how policy is developed and delivered and the how the NHS is funded. This knowledge will enhance their ability to influence key stakeholders.
- *Understanding NHS organisations* and the ways in which influence, power and authority are used.
- *Team-building skills.* These are necessary not only to get individuals in the team working together (intragroup relations) but also to develop the relationships between different teams within the organisation (intergroup relations).
- *Coping with uncertainty and stress.* Effective leaders are needed to bring about significant change, and to survive they must be able to cope in a difficult environment. However, leaders face enormous pressures and require coping strategies to ensure they are adaptable and flexible. Many programmes focus on helping individuals to ensure that there is a sensible balance between work and personal life and to maintain physical and mental health.
- *Personal skills*, such as conflict resolution, negotiation and presentation skills, can be developed.

Although some of these characteristics of leadership may be learned through formal seminars and workshops, most leadership development programmes encourage other learning approaches. These include:

- *Action learning sets* in which a group of 5–8 individuals is led by an experienced facilitator and each individual in turn uses the experiences, knowledge and expertise of others to work through problems arising from or within the organisation.
- *Networking,* which is crucial to effective leadership as it provides access to new ideas and ways of working and broadens horizons. It also helps provide support and advice from others. Networks may be both formal and informal.
- *Mentors,* who can develop dynamic relationships with individuals and assist in empowering them to discover and use their own talents. They do this by encouraging, nurturing, coaching, guiding and acting as a role model.
- *Shadowing,* in which individuals spend time with experienced, well-respected role models to learn first-hand what they do and how they work. This may be within the NHS or in other organisations. The benefits of shadowing someone from a different organisation are that it will broaden the person's outlook and highlight similarities and differences in the work environment.

- *Project work* is also used to give participants the opportunity to study an issue in depth that will help both the organisation and the individual.

The *NHS Modernisation Agency* has taken the primary role for leadership in the NHS. In April 2001 it established a Leadership Centre to take this forward. The Leadership Centre does not itself provide all leadership training but aims to identify and promote good leadership behaviour by identifying developmental opportunities to enable individuals to develop appropriate competences and skills. To this end the Centre commissions national and pilot programmes, sets standards for what is required and monitors providers. In addition the Centre works with managers to produce a more systematic approach to career development for leaders and promotes equality and diversity (DoH 2001a,b).

A specific initiative aimed at nurses is the development of the NHS Nursing Leadership Project launched in November 2001. Under the auspices of this project the Centre for the Development of Nursing Policy and Practice at Leeds University, in conjunction with the originators of Leading Empowered Organisations, in Minneapolis, USA, provided a three-day course: the *Leading Empowered Organisations (LEO) Programme*. LEO is aimed at healthcare professionals from all disciplines and all levels of expertise. It is intended to help frontline staff to effect and lead change; to enable them to develop healthy working relationships and become skilled problem-solvers and confident risk-takers (DoH 2001a,b).

A second initiative aimed at nurses is the *Royal College of Nursing Clinical Leadership Programme*. This is a patient-centred, practical needs-led programme lasting 18 months and designed to assist healthcare practitioners in the development of strategies to deal with the realities of their day-to-day practice. It requires the release of the clinical leader for 25% of their time and a local full-time facilitator is required for a group undergoing the programme. In addition, the programme provides a number of online resources relating to leadership such as leadership tools, pyschometric tests, mentoring resources and links to relevant websites. There are many more leadership development programmes available, from the well-established Kings Fund Leadership Programme to those provided locally by individual trusts, higher education establishments and other education providers.

Management versus leadership

On superficial examination it appears there is much overlap between management and leadership. It can be argued that there are commonalities and that a combination of both leadership and management abilities in an individual is helpful. However, on a deeper look at the two concepts there are significant differences. Managers have subordinates and use a set of techniques, including planning, setting objectives, organising, coordinating and implementing rules in the form of policies and procedures. They are concerned with efficiency and work by demanding, insisting, directing, convincing colleagues and encouraging cooperation. Leaders, on the other hand, have followers. They are concerned with direction issues, presenting dreams, developing cultures, exploring possibilities and analysing problems. They work by inspiring people and exploiting opportunities within the environment in which they are working.

Handy (1991) suggests that organisations whose work can be precisely described and defined and therefore carefully monitored and controlled can be managed more readily than organisations that are changing, complex and need to be flexible to meet different demands. In the former situation, managers feel more comfortable because they can be clear about boundaries, control methods and therefore results. The changing organisation requires people who can work in new ways and who can be creative, innovative and live with a degree of uncertainty. There is no doubt that for more than a decade the NHS has been rapidly changing, with new demands made on it every day. Consequently there has been an increasing value placed on leadership in healthcare, based on recognition of the changing NHS and the need to have people with the skills described above. The NHS Plan recognises that modernisation requires first-class leaders at all levels and indicates that senior experienced practitioners such as nurse consultants, modern matrons, ward sisters and charge nurses are ideally placed to take on leadership roles (DoH 2000). Whilst advanced practitioners are not specifically named in the Plan, the implication is that they too, by virtue of their expertise, will act as clinical and professional leaders. The focus on leadership development has been so extensive that there is a danger of management skills being seen as having less importance. However, the following description by Covey (1992) shows how the two go hand-in-hand and that both sets of abilities are essential. He describes management as 'having the bottom line focus – How can I best accomplish things?' and leadership as 'having the top line focus – What are the things I want to accomplish?' From this it can be seen that leadership skills are required to set the vision and management skills are required to achieve it.

Supporting leadership

People working in leadership positions give a considerable amount of personal commitment and energy and there is a danger that they become too focused on the work they are doing or the people they work with, causing their own physical, mental and social well-being to suffer. It is essential that leaders take time to keep in good shape, as well as reflect on and develop their clinical, professional and leadership practice. The advanced practitioner needs to be an effective leader, including supervision, reflection, mentorship and facilitation in their way of working.

Clinical supervision

The supervisory relationship is intended to assist supervised individuals to learn through and from their experiences, to aid personal development and effectiveness. Butterworth and Faugier (1992: 12) argue that clinical supervision is 'an exchange between practising professionals to enable the development of professional skills' that they go on to suggest has the function of 'improving skills, knowledge and support for supervisees which ultimately results in improved patient care'. The UKCC/NMC support this view, stating that clinical supervision 'brings practitioners and skilled supervisors together to reflect on practice. Supervision aims to identify solutions to problems, improve practice and increase understanding of professional issues' (NMC 2000).

Clinical supervision can provide an arena in which advanced practitioners can safely discuss their leadership activities and receive impartial advice or guidance about a proposed course of action. The advanced practitioner can also bring to the supervisory meeting experiences of particular events for discussion and analysis. Finally, supervision helps advanced practitioners to recognise the emotional and psychological demands placed on them and develop strategies for coping effectively with these. This is important because, whilst they may have followers, leaders can also find themselves feeling alone and under pressure as everyone else looks to them to provide strength and inspiration. Leaders need space in which they can acknowledge their own limitations and seek ways of dealing with these without incurring a high personal cost.

Reflection

Schön (1983) argues that the way professionals think in practice provides a way of learning that cannot be found through other sources. The realities of the practice setting differ from the standard presentations of textbooks, and practitioners have to be able to adapt theoretical knowledge, integrating this with experiences, to deal with real situations. The messier these situations are, the less likely it is that a neat, tidy, technical solution can be found. Schön (1983) proposes that by engaging in reflection, professionals are able to engage in *reflection in action*, analysing experience as it is occurring and whilst they are practising in the clinical arena. They are also able to engage in *reflection on action*, looking back on incidents that have occurred. Advanced practitioners who use reflection are better able to assess the suitability of a course of action and are more aware of their actions. Reflection helps to guard against complacency and increases the ability to see other sides to a situation.

Mentorship

A mentor is 'someone who provides an enabling relationship which facilitates another's growth and development' (Morton-Cooper & Palmer 1993). Mentorship is concerned with individual growth, development of confidence, creativity, self-awareness and fulfilment of potential, and the mentoring relationship provides teaching, coaching, counselling, sponsorship, guidance and support to achieve this. Morton-Cooper and Palmer claim the following benefits to the mentor, mentoree and the organisation concerned:

- The mentor gains personal satisfaction from assisting another's development.
- The mentoree develops job satisfaction and possibilities of advancement.
- The organisation has a satisfied, motivated workforce with positive outcomes for customers and clients.

For the advanced practitioner there are potential benefits whatever role they play.

Facilitation

Facilitation encourages personal development in a non-confrontational, flexible environment, with the facilitator acting as a learning resource. Morton-Cooper and Palmer (1993) suggest that, to promote effective learning, facilitative relationships have to be based on trust, respect and a genuine valuing of each other's abilities. They believe that this role fits well with the ethos of adult learning. These characteristics also fit well with the approaches described above in which leaders are empowering individuals and value others' contributions.

Leadership in advanced practice

If nurses working in advanced practice are to make a real difference to patients they must not only be effective practitioners but also be effective leaders and influence healthcare in different ways and at different levels. A good starting point is to be able to manage themselves.

Self-management requires advanced practitioners to be able to reflect on their working lives, their qualities and characteristics, styles and skills and to identify their strengths and weaknesses. They should consider what impact they have on the people they work with, how they need to modify or develop their knowledge, skills and behaviour to get more of what they want and how they need to develop and improve their own competence. It is also useful if they look outside their immediate area of practice and gain a better understanding of their organisation and the NHS as a whole and ask themselves how well their work contributes to the larger entity, and if it needs to change.

Clinical and professional leadership

As experienced and specialist senior nurses, advanced practitioners will have an important leadership role in clinical practice as they are likely to have the most nursing expertise in that particular field in the organisation. Their efforts will involve ensuring effective healthcare is provided for a specific group of patients or areas of practice that results in improved quality and health outcomes. This will be achieved by innovating and changing practice, through research and evaluation and providing expert advice to others inside and outside nursing. Clinical leadership should be combined with effective professional leadership, with the advanced nurse practitioner working within and across professional and organisational boundaries to influence other disciplines to help deliver better services. This will provide opportunities to encourage interprofessional and inter-agency working, working collaboratively with others, sharing knowledge and ideas and acting as an effective role model.

There are different levels at which those in advanced practice can exert influence and use both clinical and professional leadership talents.

Local level

Advanced practitioners provide both clinical and professional leadership in their own organisations. They work with colleagues in the relevant multidisciplinary teams, for example, skin cancer, rheumatology, or a community-based team. Advanced practitioners have a vision of how to improve the health of the group of patients they are responsible for and identify the health outcomes desired to meet national and international standards. They develop the nursing component of the patient care pathway and set the standard and level of care expected. They may also play a key role in coordinating contributions from other healthcare professionals working in the same and different organisations. This will require real understanding from the patient's as well as the professional perspective to ensure there is continuity of healthcare across traditional boundaries.

At local level the advanced practitioner should be a strong influence on the generic teams working in wards and departments. This involves identifying the steps required to develop excellence in nursing care for a group of patients, such as skilled assessments, research-based interventions and the competences required. The advanced practitioner ensures that training and development programmes and other learning opportunities are provided and that there is a systematic programme for audit, evaluation and monitoring.

Frequently, an advanced practitioner will work with several generic teams, for example in the case of a tissue viability and palliative care service. This type of working is dependent on collaboration with the relevant managers, finding out how they see the situation and how they feel as a basis for negotiating decisions on how to move forward. Such negotiations include being clear about what needs to be done and by whom, bringing in effective communication skills, developing team spirit and offering training, development and support.

At local level it is also important that the advanced practitioner can influence the organisation's strategy. This will require influencing the chief nurse and senior managers. The advanced practitioner should remember that the chief nurse and managers are not experts in their field and need support and advice in these specialist areas of practice. Advanced practitioners must, however, do their homework and find out the best way of engaging these individuals and presenting their ideas. This is essential in helping them to understand and actively support the vision and plan.

Leadership at local level should also involve patients, carers and the public in shaping the vision, in planning, evaluating and monitoring service provision and, if necessary, in lobbying for resources. Finding out what patients want is not easy: focus groups, patients' panels and patient story-telling are techniques that can be used in addition to the more traditional surveys and interviews.

Commissioners

A considerable amount of healthcare is commissioned by the local primary care trusts in order to meet the health needs of the local population. Advanced practitioners need to work with their multidisciplinary teams and managers to share their strategy and plan with commissioners. They have to 'buy into' the service; in other words they have to see the service as being beneficial to patients in terms of health outcomes as a priority and what patients want. The service also has to be cost-effective and affordable and fit in with the Health Improvement Programme

(HIMP) for the health economy concerned. Sometimes local patient interest and pressure groups can add weight to the argument for developing services in a particular way and they can help to shape the vision as well as to influence the commissioners.

Nationally

Advanced practitioners should use their leadership ability to influence the national agenda to ensure that strategies across the country target the best health outcomes for patients and that resources are focused on these. Those individuals with responsibility for setting the agenda rarely have as much recent experience as advanced practitioners, and they rely on getting advice from experts working in a speciality.

Raising awareness and interest in a specific area of practice can be achieved by publishing. Practitioners working in a speciality tend to write for specialist journals. Although this is useful for sharing innovative practices with other specialists it does not reach the more generalist practitioner or senior manager responsible for identifying priorities and setting the agenda. Writing for more popular clinical, professional and management journals will help to raise awareness, particularly if the article is written in a way that appeals to these groups.

It is important that people working in advanced practice make contact with colleagues in the Department of Health. There are individuals there who have a lead responsibility for most specialities in healthcare and this will not only provide an opportunity to keep up to date with the latest thinking but also create the chance to influence decisions and strategy. Professional bodies and associations of nurses working in specialist areas can also be influential in changing practices to improve standards and develop professional practice across the whole profession and health service. This requires extra commitment from nurses, who often spend some of their own time in such activities. Their collective advice, however, is often sought at different levels of the health service by those developing and planning services and by individuals working in a speciality. Advanced practitioners should also consider linking with national patients' associations, voluntary bodies and charities that are relevant to the speciality. Views of patients and carers can be helpful in developing plans and these bodies can be supportive when lobbying for support and resources.

Conclusion

For individual advanced practitioners to make a difference to patients they have to have clinical and professional expertise that is developed through education, training and experience. However, if they are to make a real difference to patient groups and the wider health economy they must be able to influence others. To do this they must be able to influence the vision and plans at different levels of the NHS, and win the hearts and minds of people they work with so that they too will support the plan and pursue the vision. This requires effective leadership and influencing abilities that can be learned and further developed throughout their careers.

? **Key questions for Chapter 6**

In your field of practice:

(1) Which styles of leadership are evident and how might these help or support the advanced practitioner?
(2) In your view should advanced practitioners combine leadership with management responsibilities?
(3) In what specific ways might the advanced practitioner provide leadership, at local and national levels?

References

Adair, J. (1984) *Action Centred Leadership*. London: McGraw-Hill.

Armstrong, M. (1994) How to be an even better manager: a complete A–Z of proven techniques. In: *Leadership*, 4th edn, pp. 173–81. London: Kogan Page.

Briggs, K.C. & Briggs Myers, I. (1989) Myers Briggs type indicators. In: *Leading in the NHS: A Practical Guide* (ed. R. Stewart). Basingstoke: Macmillan.

Butterworth, T. & Faugier, J. (1992) (eds) *Clinical Supervision and Mentorship in Nursing*. London: Chapman & Hall.

Cole, G.A. (1997) Personnel management. In: *Leadership in Organizations*, pp. 49–59. London: Letts Educational.

Covey, S.R. (1992) *The 7 Habits of Highly Effective People: Powerful Lessons in Personal Change*. London: Franklin Covey Co.

DoH (2000) *The NHS Plan: A Plan for Investment, A Plan for Reform*. London: DoH.

DoH (2001a) *Modernisation Agency, Leadership Centre*. Available at www.modernnhs.nhs.uk

DoH (2001b) *Nursing Leadership Project*. Available at www.nursingleadership.nhs.uk

Handy, C. (1991) *The Age of Unreason*. London: Century Business.

Lock, D. (1992) *Gower Handbook of Management*, 3rd edn. London: BCA/Gower.

Morton-Cooper, A. & Palmer, A. (1993) *Mentoring and Preceptorship: A Guide to Support Roles in Clinical Practice*. London: Blackwell Science.

NMC (2000) *Position Statement on Clinical Supervision for Nursing Midwifery and Health Visiting*, para. 11. London: NMC. Available at http://www.nmc-uk.org

O'Connor, C.A. (1994) *Successful Leadership in a Week*. London: Institute of Management Foundation/Hodder & Stoughton.

Plant, R. (1987) *Managing Change and Making it Stick*. London: Fontana.

Rowntree, D. (1989) *The Manager's Book of Checklists: A Practical Guide to Improving Managerial Skills*. Aldershot: Gower.

Schön, D. (1983) *The Reflective Practitioner: How Professionals Think in Action*. London: Avebury.

Waitley, D. (1994) *The New Dynamics of Winning: Gain the Mind-set of a Champion*. London: Nicholas Brealey.

Yates, M. (1999) *Leadership: Truth and Process*. Available at http://www.leader-values.com

Chapter 7

Providing a Culture of Learning for Advanced Practice Students undertaking a Master's Degree

Chris Inman

Introduction

There appears to be a consensus that advanced practitioners should be educated at master's degree level. Support for requiring this level of education in the UK is evident in the United Kingdom Central Council's documents on post-registration and in its work on higher-level practice (UKCC 1994, 2002). The American Nurses' Association, along with national bodies in other countries such as Canada, has stated that it regards a master's degree as a mandatory part of becoming an advanced practitioner because such degrees demonstrate academic progression from initial nurse education (Hamric *et al.* 2000; Locking-Cusolito 2000). In addition, the International Council of Nurses has recommended master's degrees for entry to advanced practice in all countries (ICN 2002).

This recommendation is not surprising given the requirements of the advanced nursing role. The definition of advanced practice put forward in Chapter 3 of this book makes it clear that the practitioner must demonstrate expert clinical performance complemented by a high level of interpersonal competence (see Fig. 3.1 on page 25). This competence extends into collaborative styles of working, consultancy roles and cultural expertise to challenge professional boundaries and develop practice. The advanced practitioner engages in critical and reflective practice as a basis for providing clinical and professional leadership, using sound ethical reasoning in dealing with dilemmas in care and engaging in scholarly activity that promotes an increase in nursing knowledge and skills for the benefit of the patient, the advanced practitioner, the nursing profession or all of these.

The complexity of the advanced role clearly demands a level of education commensurate with the level of responsibility involved. The question then arises as to how best to help aspiring advanced practitioners acquire the knowledge and skills required and convincingly demonstrate the wide range of competences required. This chapter presents an account of one MSc in Advanced Practice (MScAP) course at the University of Central England. The value of doing so is, first, that this programme, with an essential practice component as well as a research project, is unusual at master's level. It encapsulates perfectly the principles identified by the Quality Assurance Agency for Higher Education that stated that study at master's level should demonstrate 'a systematic understanding of knowledge, and a critical awareness of current problems and/or new insights, much of which is at, or informed by, the forefront of their academic discipline, field of study, or professional practice' (QAA 2001). This QAA statement, written after the development of the course described in this chapter, reflects the qualities and outcomes that the course team aimed to include during development and at delivery of the course.

Second, the MScAP students have a challenge not experienced by many other master's level students: that of demonstrating that they have advanced not only academically to master's level but also in their practice and that they are involved in improving care. This is not comparable to many other disciplines. For example, an arts student may be required to create, analyse and demonstrate knowledge of a sculpture or picture; the science student may test a theory by experiment, but the advanced practice student is working in a social capacity with people who, owing to illness, impairment or disability, may be vulnerable. The MScAP students have therefore to cope with a significant additional burden of practice learning that involves working with people and collaborating with other professionals to complete the master's study within the same period of time as peers from other disciplines. For the extra strand of learning and development the students need additional practice-related study time and extra practice facilitation and academic support. In essence, for the MScAP students the qualities of a professional as well as an academic are being extended, normally within a relatively short time. For this learning to be supported, the course team has created a culture of learning that fosters the students' development within and beyond the structural limits of the learning environment in the university (Abercrombie 1993). For this total quality learning 'learning organisations' need to be ready to provide time and resources to support students and staff (Lessem 1991).

Third, the NHS Plan (DoH 2000) and related policy documents (DoH 1999) provide senior nurses and midwives with opportunities to increase their autonomy by becoming involved with more comprehensive assessments, investigations and treatments, including some prescribing rights. These changes have been influenced by a massive and continuing reduction in junior doctors' hours during the past decade and the Nursing and Midwifery Council's new Code of Professional Conduct that reflects values that are now common for health professionals in the UK (NMC 2002). Such factors, combined with the higher health expectations of patients, have led to a shortfall in the number of health professionals who can provide high standard, effective healthcare. Advanced practitioners are now needed as never before to use their expertise in providing direct care, particularly to those who might otherwise have limited access to health services.

This chapter begins by setting the scene with an overview of the MScAP course but the main focus is on the strategy used to enable students to develop their skills in and for practice, with a particular focus on advanced health assessment. The modules on advanced health assessment are outlined. These modules are initially classroom-based but the students are then required to apply their learning in their practice setting under the supervision of practice facilitators who assess their progress. The second part of the chapter presents a discussion of the strategies employed to enable students to develop the skills required for critical practice through, for example, small working groups. The chapter closes with a consideration of some of the obstacles that can prevent students from making the progress required.

The aim and structure of the course

The MScAP contains a mixture of compulsory and optional modules (Table 7.1). Compulsory modules, including Advanced Health Assessment, Research, and Leadership, cover those topics deemed essential for every advanced practitioner. Optional modules are specific, linked either to particular fields of practice or topic areas that the individual may wish to study in more depth. There are three possible exit points:

- Postgraduate certificate attained on completing four modules, one of which is selected from the list of optional topics.
- Postgraduate diploma awarded on completing eight modules, two of which are selected from the list of optional topics.
- The master's degree which is awarded on completion of a series of multi-disciplinary research workshops and a dissertation or clinical pathway research project (Table 7.1).

The course team, in consultation with stakeholders, selected the course modules. These stakeholders included practitioners from many different fields of nursing, midwifery, members of professions allied to medicine, and physicians. NHS service users, managers and officials were also consulted.

Applicants to the course must have a minimum of three years in post-registration practice, but the majority easily exceed this. Those without a degree or the equivalent are required to complete some pre-course study regardless of experience and seniority. This course includes mandatory physiology at CATs level two or three and research methods at CATs level three. Other modules may also be included depending on the individual's education and experience. Consequently, entry to the course may take some time, but most applicants realise the value of the preparation as they progress through the master's course.

Table 7.1 The MSc in Advanced Practice course.

Postgraduate certificate modules	Postgraduate diploma modules	Master's degree
Analysis of Advanced Practice	Research Methods	Multidisciplinary research workshops
Advanced Health Assessment (1)	Advanced Health Assessment (2)	
Leadership and Management of Change	Advanced Practicum	Dissertation or clinical pathway project
Optional module 1	Optional module 2	

Optional module topics
Children-critical Perspectives
Current Issues in Public Health
Economic and Policy Issues
Ethical and Legal Issues
Midwifery
Teaching and Guidance
Women's Health

Advanced health assessment

Three of the modules address advanced health assessments. A double Advanced Health Assessment (AHA) module is taught in the University and these two modules together carry a total of 300 notional study hours, with a minimum of 60 hours being spent in direct teaching contact time in classroom/practical room settings. The Advanced Practicum module is the third, and this facilitates the application of the AHA university teaching to the students' own practice populations and settings. The Advanced Practicum module counts as a double module with a notional 300 study/application hours because the practice development is crucial and needs adequate time.

The term 'practicum' was coined by Schön (1983). He placed a high value on intuition and the ability of professionals to draw on practice experiences and advocated the use of 'an epistemology of practice implicit in the artistic, intuitive processes which some practitioners do bring to situations of uncertainty, instability, uniqueness, and value conflict' (p. 49). Schön's passion for the artistic and intuitive stemmed from his rejection of the positivism and technical rationality on which medicine was then based. However, training for the medical professional is no longer dominated by positivism but involves substantial teaching of more naturalistic methodologies that can include narrative-based medical health assessment, an approach rarely considered by medical practitioners or their teachers when Schön was developing his theories in the 1980s. Moreover, in teaching physical assessment to experienced health professionals, the most proficient practitioner readily available in the UK is the medical practitioner.

Consequently, a doctor is employed on the MScAP course to teach in the Advanced Practicum module. The doctor focuses on physical assessment, beginning with a separate systems approach but culminating with a whole head-to-toe physical assessment where all the body systems are considered. The rationale for carrying out a full physical assessment, as opposed to just observing the patient, is discussed with reference to each system, the chief complaint, taking a comprehensive past and present history. This is followed by the information regarding approaches to physically assessing a particular system. A demonstration, in which students act as models follows with the doctor talking through the examination and the communication needed to gain the 'patient's' cooperation. All students then practise assessing that physical system, normally in groups of three or four, whilst the doctor and nurse lecturers guide and prompt the students. On the same day, the formal teaching is followed at a more relaxed pace by a practice application session. For this, students are encouraged to practise on one another the physical assessment that they have earlier covered with the medical practitioner, working in small groups with lecturers to support and supervise (Griffiths 1999). During this time the students can, if they wish, also watch and critique the Bates Physical Assessment tapes (Bates 1995). These twenty-minute videotapes address each system and include a review of the anatomy.

The doctor's sessions alternate with classes led by a physiologist who prepares the students for the next AHA session. This preparation helps to refresh the students' knowledge and understanding and ensures that they are building onto and revising their knowledge of the system, and seeking new and established research and theory relating to the physiology. Other lecturing that complements the medical practitioners' and physiologists' session includes interpreting X-rays, pharmacology, critical incidents, critical thinking and decision-making, risk assessment and competences. Students are introduced to a range of models for physical health assessment to help them select the most appropriate tools for their field of practice (see, for example, Fuller & Schaller-Ayres 1994; Bates 1995; Epstein *et al.* 1997; Seidal *et al.* 1999; and models such as Problem Orientated Medical Record (POMR) and Subjective Objective Assessment Plan (SOAP)).

The AHA modules are taught throughout the first academic year. The taught element begins at the start of the course and the practice-related element, the Advanced Practicum, is completed and documented by the end of the postgraduate diploma, thus allowing students the entire period of the course for structured practice and support. The aim is to enable the student to gain the maximum amount of practice experience possible and provide adequate time for development, rather than try to complete the experience quickly to meet a course deadline.

The practice application of AHAs

Opportunities for the students to practise advanced health assessments in their own workplace settings are seen to be an essential element of development. Applicants to the course are required to identify potential practice facilitator(s). Places are not given to those who do not have hands-on involvement with patients or who lack the support of facilitators, managers and the multiprofessional team. A minimum of two practice facilitators is normally required. One supports the development of physical advanced health assessment skills and the other focuses on role and professional development for the student. A doctor or an experienced advanced practitioner who graduated from an earlier master's course is normally the most suitable facilitator to support the development of physical assessment skills. Medical facilitators who have influential positions in a directorate are particularly valuable since they will then have full knowledge of the way the student's skills are being developed. They also have an understanding of the way services are structured that helps them to identify aspects of service where an advanced practitioner could make a significant impact on improving care. A senior nurse/midwifery manager or experienced advanced practitioner is often an excellent facilitator for role and contract/job description professional development. This person may also be able to support the student in other ways such as assessing the health needs of a population, care pathway development and evaluation.

The practice health assessment facilitators are asked to attend a meeting with the module coordinator and student to help them to prepare for their role. During the meeting the facilitators can ask questions and clarify issues. The course director talks the student and facilitator through the practice profile documentation that supports the student's learning. The student's action plan and possible learning experience and critical incident analyses are discussed. The other University-assessed assignments are explained, in particular those related to AHAs. The facilitator might be able to support the student in identifying a suitable focus for assignments to deepen their learning and by passing on any new supporting literature they come across. All of this is intended to ensure that the facilitators are gaining an understanding of their role and developing a commitment to support the student.

The practice profile element of the course involves all the qualities of student-centred learning (Cowan 1998). Each student has a practice profile that allows documentation of practice development. This includes an initial and revised action plan that the student is responsible for negotiating and documenting with the practice facilitators. The learning identified in this plan should be highly relevant to what is needed for practice development and what is of interest to the student. A competence checklist is also integrated into the practice profile and this includes a midway and summative self- and facilitator assessment. Critical incident analysis is also required. Finally the student is required to write a reflective summary of the practice experience.

Assessing the AHA modules

Assessment of practice takes two forms with several separate elements within each. These include written assignments – such as an individual patient case study and the macro health assessment of a population – that are needed to help demonstrate a strong knowledge base and critical thinking and reflection alongside strategies for assessing practice that include a learning contract and regular assessment by the facilitator. To date, external examiners have been satisfied with the evidence presented from the current methods. However, the course team is considering introducing observed structured clinical examinations as described by Brown (1999), particularly if extended prescribing is made available as an optional module.

Students' need time to practise and reflect on newly acquired knowledge and skills involved in AHAs without being under pressure. Furthermore, ongoing and eventually summative self-assessment is required, as well as facilitator assessment and feedback. Cowan (1998) contests Boud's (1995) use of the term 'self-assessment', which Cowan argues refers to self-evaluation and is concerned with comparing performance with a set of standards. Using Cowan's definitions the MScAP students are involved with self-evaluation of process, in their ongoing and midway assessment. They are also engaged in self-assessment of outcome alongside their facilitators for their summative assessment when a judgement of pass or fail needs to be made (Cowan 1998). A completed copy of the practice profile is submitted to the module coordinator for scrutiny and comment and is then sent to the external examiner.

Supporting the development of critical practice

Early in the course a variety of models and structures to support critiquing are provided and discussed. These are focused on analysing research methodologies or other evidence used to evaluate practice to encourage the students to discriminate intelligently (Girot 1995). The emphases are on developing a critical approach to avoid over-reliance on the written text, and guiding students to question and challenge normal practice and to examine the underlying assumptions (Ramsden 1999). Critical thinking skills are also needed in relation to advanced health assessment and will become essential to support clinical judgements and decision-making, facilitating the development of 'intellectual independence and relativistic reasoning' in students to help them to think like a clinician as well as a nurse/midwife (Eizenberg 1988; Seidel *et al.* 1999).

Students are encouraged to analyse materials alone, selecting approaches that best suit their needs, and to discuss the outcomes in small workshop groups. This provides opportunities for students to present arguments and justify their conclusions in front of their peers. This type of teaching needs managing carefully to develop group relationships, group support and cohesion (Griffiths 1999). Positive facilitation provides an enjoyable interactive, cognitive and affective learning situation where the students collaborate to improve the learning environment – all skills that they can carry forward to support them in lifelong learning. The range of skills needed for group learning includes:

- Developing personal time-management skills to set time aside for the course
- In-depth reading, responding to, thinking about and summarising the content
- Working collaboratively in diverse groups of practitioners to negotiate priorities to present to the whole group of students
- Presentation skills, 'off the cuff' maybe using a whiteboard, without preparation time to produce refined overheads
- Justifying decisions and answering questions from peers
- Providing written, constructive feedback for peer students on their performances.

The intention is to provide students, throughout the course, with a range of tools and opportunities in a relatively non-threatening environment in preparation for more formal and structured presentations in both the University and the workplace, for example to medical facilitators or trust committees. For such activities it is essential that the students are accurate, systematic and analytical, able to discuss and negotiate a plan of care and treatment with the patient, and are able to justify this plan to the senior heath professional who is likely to be a practitioner of some seniority.

One aspect of the theoretical and knowledge teaching is the requirement that students relate their practice development to the theoretical material consistently. Theoretical material includes policy documents. Conversely, the theoretical material needs to be related to their practice. Evidence of this linking is required in all written assignments, in seminar work and in documentation related to practice development. The requirement for practice application is developed to encourage students to integrate the theoretical and practice-based material. None find this easy, especially early in the course, but the consistency for this requirement throughout the programme of modules helps most students to internalise this skill as they progress through the course.

In educational terms, Biggs (1999) provides an analysis of deep and surface learning. The ideal aim for deep learning is to encourage the students from the outset to retain the enthusiasm and deep interest in their development that most express when applying for the course; to build onto, deepen and expand existing knowledge by working from first principles and tracking valuable theories and concepts back to their seminal sources. Conversely, the intention is to avoid surface learning where students devote insufficient time to developing their knowledge base and fail to understand essential concepts and theories at a deep level. The teachers avoid teaching disparate 'facts' out of context; avoid allowing insufficient time for the students to engage in learning so they develop low expectations of success (Biggs 1999:14). This deep approach to learning is the ideal. For some students it is achieved and provides a highly satisfying learning experience. It supports role advancement and enables them to take responsibility for more holistic care and greater involvement for evaluating improved care. It can also involve taking professional/career risks, greater responsibility and being prepared to be at the cutting edge of the advancement of their profession.

The impact of external influences on student learning

For a significant number of students the learning satisfaction anticipated is jeopardised by the emergence of unforeseen barriers that can interrupt studying temporarily and occasionally permanently. These barriers can arise from work pressures and/or from changes in family circumstances – what might be broadly referred to as 'life events'. They can constitute, at best, a significant interruption if they occur separately, but if work and family changes occur in conjunction the barrier to student learning can prove insurmountable. This aspect of learning is rarely addressed in the literature relating to supporting learning in higher education. Being able to trust the course director and team to support them through difficult times can make the difference between attrition and slight delay in progress for the student.

The origin of work barriers is complex. It can include the student feeling secure as a practitioner at work and insecure, uncertain and challenged at university, necessitating support in moving between two very different environments. It can also be due to professional barriers emerging at work, maybe even professional jealousy that seems to arise more often from colleagues of the same profession than from medical staff or from other professionals allied to medicine. Alternatively, it can be due to inadequate time being available for professional clinical development and study. Whilst, in most cases, managers have agreed to support the student with time and/or financial help during the course, pressure from managers for students to sacrifice study time and practice development time, even the formal teaching time in university, has gradually increased. Students on the course are already senior nurses and thus key figures for the increasing amount of quality reviews for the National Service Framework and other standard reviews that have appeared in the past few years.

The other significant influence on learning is the students' personal life. Family might, for some students, be providing immeasurable significant support. Other students may suffer a compromised learning experience because of family. Another challenge, the extent of which is not normally anticipated, is the change experienced in the students' personal development and the effect on their private lives. When it is suggested to students that they may be altered by undertaking master's level study they tend to deny this possibility. But this has parallels with the 'educating Rita' scenario and can have a profound effect on personal relationships.

Almost all students require support at some stage of their development. It is fortunate that numbers are small, normally about 20 in each year-group. In the past students have been allocated personal tutors but these people were rarely accessed by the student, the reason being that because of the small numbers the course director knows most students quite well and the students relate to her, knowing she is also responsible for the management of the course and has a keen interest in their progress. It is recognised that the course director may not, however, be a student's first or best choice for support. In acknowledgement of this students are given contact details of a wide variety of academic and administrative staff. This means students are empowered to access support from people with appropriate knowledge and skills or in whom they have most confidence.

Advanced practitioners as professionals

Whilst this chapter cannot include in-depth analysis of the extensive literature regarding what constitutes a profession, neither can this related issue be completely omitted. Advanced practice graduates almost always practise much more independently than prior to the course. They normally undertake roles that involve increased responsibility because of the skills they have developed. A synopsis of the literature on professions can be found in Eraut (1994). Central to professionalism and the recognition of powerful professions such as medicine and law is the existence of a professional knowledge base that encompasses knowledge and competence. Professional knowledge is a complex issue. Eraut (1994) states that it encompasses many different qualities, some of which are quite esoteric and difficult to relate to professional practice. These include tacit knowledge that cannot be articulated fully, and explicit knowledge, which is not used and remains 'in store'. This is pertinent for educating the MScAP student. Boore (1996) suggests that it is difficult to define a body of knowledge for nursing because of the need to draw on associated disciplines such as sociology, psychology and physiology. This view seems less significant in the new millennium as it is recognised that the education and knowledge base of other previously narrow professional disciplines, including doctors, needs to be much more eclectic and include substantial teaching from many of the same disciplines as nursing. For advanced practitioners in nursing and midwifery the body of knowledge has been defined clearly and by many authors, including Hamric (2000) and McGee and Castledine (this volume). Whilst variations are evident within the frameworks, the consensus that emerges suggests that at an advanced level it is not difficult to define the body of knowledge. It is, however, important to be selective so that what is included in a master's course supports effective learning.

Professions have in the past been self-regulating, setting their own standards to protect the public against 'incompetence, carelessness and exploitation' (Eraut 1994: 2). They have enjoyed statutory protection of their status by governments and protection of their profession from any potential competing professional group, a so-called sheltered market position. This is in exchange for their services in maintaining the citizens, in this instance in health. In the past, nursing and midwifery have not enjoyed the autonomy of full professional recognition that the medical profession has because government and doctors have influenced nurses' and midwives' educational standards, practice boundaries and working conditions. To end on a more positive note, nursing and midwifery do, however, fulfil many features of professionalism. For example, the existence of a code of professional conduct and associated disciplinary procedures (NMC 2002).

Conclusion

This chapter has provided an overview of some of the issues related to running an MSc in Advanced Practice course. A heavy focus has been placed on the practice component because this aspect is normally the reason for students selecting the course. It is, however, also this aspect that puts significant additional pressure on the students. Related to this is the critical thinking and reflection needed for advanced health assessments and academic work. Professional issues are central to advanced practice and these have also been raised briefly in this chapter. The final word should go to a comment made by a graduate in a follow-up survey. Her view was: 'I feel that working as an advanced practitioner is more about attitude, innovation, forward thinking and leading all aspects of my work, than a title alone would suggest.'

? **Key questions for Chapter 7**

In your field of practice:

(1) In what ways might advanced health assessments be of benefit to patients?
(2) What are the advantages and disadvantages of making an observed structured clinical examination mandatory for nurses learning to undertake advanced health assessments?
(3) What factors will need to be addressed in your workplace to allow nurses who conduct advanced health assessments to:
    (a) make and receive referrals to other professionals?
    (b) order investigations?

References

Abercrombie, M.L.J. (1993) *The Human Nature of Learning: Selections From the Work of Ed Nias.* Buckingham: SRHE/Open University Press.

Bates, B. (1995) *A Guide to Physical Examination and History Taking.* Philadelphia: Lippincott (videotape).

Biggs, J. (1999) *Teaching for Quality Learning in University.* Buckingham: SRHE/Open University Press.

Bickley, L.S. (1999) *Bates' Guide to Physical Examination and History Taking,* 7th edn. Philadelphia: Lippincott.

Boore, J. (1996) Postgraduate education in nursing: a case study. *Journal of Advanced Nursing,* 23: 620–29.

Boud, D. (1995) *Enhancing Learning through Self Assessment.* London: Kogan Page.

Brown, S. (1999) Assessing practice. In: *Assessment Matters in Higher Education* (eds S. Brown and A. Glasner). Buckingham: SRHE/Open University Press.

Cowan, J. (1998) *On Becoming an Innovative University Teacher.* Buckingham: Open University Press.

DoH (1999) *Making a Difference: Strengthening the Nursing, Midwifery and Health Visiting Contribution to Health and Healthcare.* London: DoH.

DoH (2000) *The NHS Plan: A Plan for Investment, A Plan for Reform.* London: DoH.

Eizenberg, N. (1988) Approaches to learning anatomy: developing a programme for pre-clinical medical students. In: *Improving Learning New Perspectives* (ed. P. Ramsden). London: Kogan Page.

Epstein, O., Perkin, G.D., de Bono, D.P. & Cookson, J. (1997) *Clinical Examination,* 2nd edn. London: Mosby.

Eraut, M. (1994) *Developing Professional Knowledge and Competence.* London: Falmer Press.

Fuller, J. & Schaller-Ayres, J. (1994) *Health Assessment: A Nursing Approach,* 2nd edn. Philadelphia: Lippincott.

Girot, E.A. (1995) Preparing the practitioner for advanced academic study: the development of critical thinking. *Journal of Advanced Nursing,* 21: 387–94.

Grant, C., Nicholas, R., Moore, L. & Salisbury, C. (2002) An observational study of quality of care in walk-in centres with general practice and NHS Direct using standardised patients. *British Medical Journal,* 324: 1556–9.

Griffiths, S. (1999) Teaching and learning in small groups. In: *A Handbook for Teaching and Learning in Higher Education: Enhancing Academic Practice* (Eds H. Fry, S. Ketteridge & S. Marshall). London: Kogan Page.

Hamric, A., Spross, J. & Hanson, C. (eds) (2000) *Advanced Nursing Practice: An Integrative Approach*, 2nd edn. Philadelphia: W.B. Saunders.

Horrocks, S., Anderson, E. & Salisbury, C. (2002) Systematic review of whether nurse practitioners in primary care provide equivalent care to doctors. London: British Medical Association.

Lessem, R. (1991) *Total Quality Learning*. Oxford: Blackwell Publishing.

Locking-Cusolito, H. (2000) Advanced practice nurses and their role in nephrology settings. *Nephrology Nursing Journal*, 27 (2): 245–7.

NMC (2002) *Code of Professional Conduct*. London: NMC.

QAA (2001) http://www.qaa.ac.uk/crntwork/nqf/ewni2001/ewni2001_textonly.htm

Quasim, A., Malpass, K. O'Gorman, D.J. & Heber, M.E. (2002) Quality improvement report: safety and efficacy of nurse-initiated thrombolysis in patients with acute myocardial infarction. *British Medical Journal*, 324: 1328–31.

Ramsden, P. (1999) *Learning to Teach in Higher Education*. London: Routledge.

Schön, D. (1983) *The Reflective Practitioner: How Professionals Think in Action*. London: Avebury.

Seidel, H.M., Ball, J.W., Dains, J.E. & Benidict, G.W. (1999) *Mosby Guide to Physical Examination*, 4th edn. St Louis: Mosby.

UKCC (1994) *The Future of Professional Practice – The Council's Standards for Education and Practice following Registration*. London: UKCC.

UKCC (2002) *Report of the Higher Level of Practice Pilot and Project*. London: UKCC.

Chapter 8

Advanced Health Assessment

Paula McGee

Introduction

The ability to assess is a key nursing skill that enables practitioners to gather relevant information about patients as a basis for the individualised planning, delivery and evaluation of care. The nature of a nursing assessment depends on a number of factors that include the health problems experienced by the patient, whether that person is presenting for the first time or has previously received care, and the nurse's knowledge and skill. This chapter begins with a case study that provides a basis for the discussion of the nature of nursing assessment using broad theoretical frameworks that enable any practitioner to gather information about patients as part of implementing the process of nursing. The second part of the chapter focuses on the type of assessment required in advanced practice. It begins with a definition of this level of advanced assessment and discusses a range of factors that may influence the direction taken by the assessor. These include the patient's sex, age and culture as well as communication issues and the nature of the presenting problem. The case study is extended to examine three forms of assessment: database, problem-oriented/follow-up, and emergency. The chapter closes with a discussion of the outcomes of such assessment, with particular reference to the formulation of nursing diagnoses and the ways in which these differ from those made by doctors.

Emergency assessment in professional practice

Marcia Williams, aged 18, has suffered from asthma all her life and has come to the accident and emergency department because she has become increasingly short of breath during the past three days and is feeling very unwell. The triage staff nurse conducts an assessment based on one of the common theoretical frameworks currently in use (Table 8.1). This framework provides a guide for assessment that can become quite detailed, but on this occasion the nurse focuses only on Marcia's immediate problems. Performing an assessment involves gathering information about the patient's current health, using a mixture of observation, measurement and semistructured interviewing. Thus the nurse observes Marcia's breathing, noting that she is breathless following her walk from the waiting area to the consulting room. The nurse also observes that Marcia is still breathless when sitting down, is breathing through her mouth and has to pause for breath several times whilst trying to explain

Table 8.1 Nursing assessment using the activities of living (Roper *et al.* 1990).

Activities of living	Initial assessment
Breathing	*Observations*: Patient is breathless and wheezing even whilst sitting down. She is using her auxiliary muscles of respiration and is breathing through her mouth. *Patients states*: She had a cold last week and that it 'went to her chest'. Marcia states that she has a cough and is bringing up 'green stuff'. Asthma is normally controlled with inhaled medication: salbutamol 400 micrograms as required and beclamethasone 200 micrograms twice daily. Marcia says she has been using these regularly but has not experienced the usual relief of symptoms. *Measurement*: She is unable to register a peak flow recording. Her previous score on routine review was 350 l/min. Her respiratory rate is rapid at 25 breaths per minute. Pulse oximetry shows saturation of 87%.
Communicating	*Observations*: Is unable to speak a sentence without pausing for breath but is able to explain her current problem.
Eating and drinking	*Patient states*: She has not eaten for the last three days but has been taking fluids. *Observations*: Lips are dry and cracked. Tongue is coated.
Mobilising	*Observations*: Breathless on exertion such as walking from the waiting area. *Patients states*: Friends brought her by car to the accident and emergency department as she felt too breathless to catch the bus.
Sleeping	*Patient states*: She has not been sleeping well even though she feels tired. She has four pillows on the bed at present instead of her usual two. She wakes several times a night feeling breathless and coughing.
Maintaining body temperature	*Measurement*: Temperature 39.7°C, pulse 115/minute. Skin is warm and appears flushed. *Patient states*: that she has been experiencing episodes of shivering, when she feels very cold.

her problem. The nurse measures Marcia's temperature, which is 39.7°C, pulse rate, which is 155/min, respiration rate which is 25 breaths per minute, and blood gas levels using pulse oximetry. The nurse also attempts to measure her peak flow but Marcia is unable to register a score. Finally the nurse asks Marcia some questions, which reveal that she has a history of a cold, a productive cough with green sputum and may have been experiencing rigors. Asking such questions requires that the nurse has well-developed interpersonal skills that not only facilitate exploration of the patient's problems but also underpin subsequent therapeutic relationships.

Assessment is the first stage in the nursing process, a decision-making pathway that provides a rational basis for the identification of the patient's problems followed by the planning, delivery and evaluation of nursing care. In this instance the triage nurse correctly identifies Marcia's main problem as an acute exacerbation of her asthma triggered by a chest infection. Recognition of this problem enables the nurse to identify appropriate nursing interventions and initiate care, for example in terms of ensuring that Marcia understands what is happening, is constantly observed for any sign of deterioration and is made as comfortable as possible. However, it is also clear that this care is not sufficient and that more advanced knowledge and skills are required, including those needed to conduct a physical examination, measurement of blood gas levels and microbiological examination of sputum, the administration of salbutamol via a nebuliser with further monitoring of peak flow and commencement of a course of antibiotics. Speedy and effective intervention is vital as most complications arise because of undertreatment or failure to appreciate the severity of the situation (Rees & Kanabar 2000). Thus Marcia may be disadvantaged by having to wait to see other health professionals.

Given the acute nature of Marcia's condition, the triage nurse quite rightly decided to concentrate on her most serious problem. The staff nurse's assessment was competent and accurate: important considerations in an emergency situation. However, the range and type of data collected in this instance is very narrow and provides no information about Marcia's daily life and the physical, psychological and social factors that may affect the management of her asthma or contribute to other problems. For example, it is not clear how much Marcia knows and understands about asthma or why friends, rather than a parent, accompany her. Such information could be obtained from a full nursing assessment that would provide a detailed account of Marcia's present and past health. In addition, Marcia should have received regular reassessments aimed at reviewing her asthma management. Once the acute episode has resolved a detailed health assessment will be needed in order to clarify the help and support Marcia needs.

An expanded concept of health

The amount of detail required in an assessment has both broadened and increased as ideas about the nature of health have changed. Health is now regarded as more than the absence of illness, as a dynamic state, in which the individual responds and adapts to challenges, rather than a continuum. The individuality of each person means that everyone will respond to challenges in a unique way aimed at maintaining and preserving well-being. Inability to respond and cope effectively may result in illness (Roy 1984). Health is, therefore, an individual experience rather than a single uniform state and it is possible to have a chronic condition, such as asthma, or a disability, and have a healthy life punctuated by episodes of ill health. Ideas about health must be based not only on how the individual is now but also on what that person may become in the future. Thinking about health requires the conceptualisation of multiple possibilities based on knowledge of the individual as a whole entity. A holistic approach to health is based on the recognition of the complexity of human existence and the diverse demands placed on individuals. In this context, health emerges as one of several, possibly competing, priorities, and health work becomes a process of enabling others to achieve what they regard as important and meaningful by helping them to manage or overcome obstacles (Seedhouse 1991).

Whilst Marcia needs immediate treatment for her chest infection, a holistic review of her health will help to create a more detailed picture of her present circumstances and the potential of these to affect her future, either positively or negatively. It is this holistic and detailed approach that characterises advanced health assessment. Cohen *et al.* (1998) liken this assessment to a mystery story in which the investigator detects and pursues clues that are then used to construct an explanation of events. In advanced health assessment the nurse collects a wide variety of data, drawing on both the individual's accounts of health and illness experiences and physical examination. This information is then collated and assessed against an extensive clinical knowledge base in order to formulate appropriate nursing diagnoses as a basis for nursing intervention tailored to the individual's needs (Jarvis 2000).

This emphasis on nursing diagnoses and intervention is important because the intention is to enhance the scope of nursing practice rather than take on medical roles. Several theorists have noted the similarities between the nursing process (Fig. 8.1) and what is frequently referred to as the 'traditional medical model' (Fig. 8.2) (see, for example, Dunphy & Winland-Brown 1998; McGee 1998). Both are based on the notion of a rational, scientific approach to practice. The *medical model* requires the doctor to collect information from the patient through interviewing, physical examination and

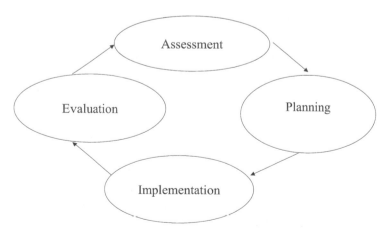

Fig. 8.1   The nursing process.

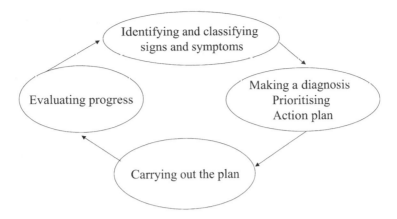

Fig. 8.2   The medical model.

scientific investigations such as blood analysis. The object is to classify information and differentiate the possible explanations for the patient's problems. From this a medical diagnosis is made on the basis of which the doctor can prioritise, select appropriate treatment and formulate an action plan. The effect of the plan is then evaluated and reformulated in the light of the patient's progress. In a similar way, the *nursing process* requires the nurse to collect information from the patient by asking questions about factors such as lifestyle, daily living activities and social background, observing physical signs such as skin integrity and making relevant measurements such as blood pressure. From this information the nurse identifies and prioritises the patient's problems as a basis for constructing an action plan in which nursing inventions are directed towards specified and individual goals. The effectiveness of this plan is then evaluated and the patient's situation is reassessed.

The introduction of the nursing process took place in the late 1960s and early 1970s at a time when nursing was attempting to reconceptualise itself as a scientifically based profession with its own body of knowledge with a rational basis for its activities. Inherent in this was a determination to achieve professional autonomy and dispense with traditional notions of subservience to medicine by taking control of domains of patient provision that were the legitimate province of the nurse. It was perhaps inevitable that nursing should borrow from medicine strategies that were both effective and regarded by doctors as reliable and appropriate.

However, after more than 30 years, it is reasonable to ask whether the nursing process still meets the needs of modern professional practice and how useful it is in relation to the current, expanded concept of health and notions of nursing care. Leininger (1984: 3) proposes that 'care is the essence and the central unifying and dominant domain to characterise nursing. Care has always been postulated to be an essential human need for the full development, health maintenance and survival of human beings in all world cultures.' She identifies three forms of care: folk, professional and nursing. Folk care is that arising from the knowledge, skill and traditions of a specific community and is thus culturally based. Professional care is that based on scientific knowledge and technological resources. Nursing care draws on both professional and folk care and integrates these with its own knowledge and skills.

Care and caring activities matter greatly because they place value on other people rather than the self. Care provides a basis for connection with others, of giving and receiving in a mutually beneficial way (Benner & Wrubel 1989). In nursing, such connections provide opportunities for specific types of care such as facilitating comfort or ensuring a peaceful death. Without care, such comfort, dignity and so on cannot occur because both patients and nurses are devalued and thus dehumanised (Benner & Wrubel 1989; Benner *et al.* 1996). This emphasis on care represents a new direction in nursing because, traditionally, nurses were taught to suppress their feelings and not to engage with patients as people (Menzies 1970; Dunlop 1986). Placing care at the centre of nursing has overturned that and altered the nature of the nurse–patient relationship. Nursing is no longer trying to prove that it is an independent profession. It has developed considerably to meet the complex healthcare needs of the twenty-first century and it is, therefore, appropriate to question whether an approach to practice based on scientific rationalism is still helpful, particularly in the context of advanced practice.

The total health assessment

This type of assessment provides a basis for the advanced practitioner to demonstrate a high level of expertise gathering information, synthesising this with an expert clinical knowledge base in order to meet healthcare needs which may be individual-, family- or community-based. A complete health assessment will involve the construction of a total health database as a foundation for both interventions and future reviews. There are two parts to this database: the health history and the physical examination (Table 8.2).

Details of the health history are acquired by interviewing the patient using a person-centred approach characterised by 'an appreciation for the uniqueness of the individuals involved [the nurse and the patient] and attention to the patient's concerns' (Spross *et al.* 2000: 195). This means that the advanced practitioner enables the patient

Table 8.2   The total health assessment.

Biographical data
General practitioner
Source of referral
Next of kin/emergency contact
Reason for seeking healthcare
History of present problem

Contd.

Table 8.2   *Contd.*

Past health history
   Serious illnesses
   Childhood illnesses
   Operations
   Travel history
   Mental health history
   Prescribed medications
   Over-the-counter medications used
   Communicable diseases
   Allergies
   Injuries/accidents
   Immunisations
   Blood transfusions

Developmental history
   Height and weight
   Breast development
   Menstrual cycle
   Sexual activity
   Pregnancy

Family health history
Work environment
Home environment
Leisure activities
Significant relationships

Review of body systems
   General appearance
   Neurological
   Eyes
   Ears
   Nose and sinuses
   Mouth and throat
   Respiratory
   Cardiovascular
   Gastrointestinal
   Urinary
   Musculoskeletal
   Reproductive
   Endocrine
   Haematological

Laboratory investigations
X-rays, scans etc.

to tell their story by conveying a genuine positive regard. The advanced practitioner is able to avoid making assumptions about the patient's problems or needs and listens attentively to what is being said. Story-telling is an art form, in which events can be recounted and interpreted in a process of negotiation with the listener for whom the story-teller provides something that, in the context of advanced health assessment, is informative and meaningful (Livo & Rietz 1986; Sandelowski 1996). The patient's story provides insight into that person's past and present experiences of health, their perceptions and understandings of their current health problems, and the psychological and social context in which these problems have arisen. Whilst listening to such stories, advanced practitioners reflect on their clinical and professional knowledge, synthesising this with the new information, summarising and recapping to clarify their understanding. In so doing the advanced practitioner creates a vocabulary of precedents that form the basis of patient-centred care.

Listening in this way brings a fresh understanding to the information Marcia has given the triage nurse. Marcia told the nurse she had a cold last week and that it 'went to her chest'. She now has a cough and is bringing up 'green stuff'. She has been using her inhalers regularly but has not experienced the usual relief of symptoms. She has not been sleeping well even though she feels tired. She has four pillows on the bed at present instead of her usual two. She has been waking several times a night feeling breathless and coughing, and has been experiencing episodes of shivering when she feels very cold. This account demonstrates the three essential elements of a story: *orientation* or beginning, *complication* in which events take place, and *evaluation* in which the outcome of events is made clear (Bell 1988). The orientation phase sets the scene: Marcia had a cold. The advanced practitioner synthesises this information with clinical knowledge about asthma, recognising that minor infections such as colds can aggravate symptoms. This raises questions in the nurse's mind about the context in which Marcia believes that she caught the cold and how much she understands about managing her asthma during such infections. In the complication phase it becomes clear that Marcia has not been sleeping well, has been experiencing breathlessness and has had a temperature. For the advanced nurse practitioner this information raises questions about the extent of the infection and the need for physical examination, Marcia's previous history of chest infections and her response to treatment as well as her state of hydration and ability to engage in self-care. Finally, the evaluation reveals that she has a productive cough that raises questions for the nurse about obtaining a sputum specimen and antibiotic therapy.

This account also demonstrates that patients may initially present their stories in highly compressed forms that may lead the less experienced practitioner to make assumptions. For example, from the triage nurse's account it would be reasonable to assume that Marcia has sought help from the accident and emergency department because she is severely breathless, but that would not explain why she has not consulted her general practitioner or why she did not seek help as soon as symptoms arose. Thus in synthesising Marcia's initial story with clinical knowledge the advanced practitioner is able to recognise the potential importance of each item of information. Patients rarely tell their stories in the straightforward manner of textbooks and no two individuals will have the same story to tell. The advanced practitioner must, therefore, be able to use the skills of reflection at the same time as listening to the patient in order to enable that person to provide a richer, more detailed account of current and past events (Table 8.2).

This verbal story is complemented by physical information (Table 8.2). The triage nurse has observed that Marcia is breathless and wheezing even whilst sitting down. She is using her auxiliary muscles of respiration and is breathing through her mouth. Her lips are dry and cracked and her tongue is coated. She is unable to register a peak flow recording. Her respiratory rate is rapid at 25 breaths per minute. Pulse oximetry shows saturation of 87%. She is unable to speak a sentence without pausing for breath and is breathless on exertion such as walking from the waiting area. The advanced practitioner is able to expand on this picture by using a range of physical examination skills that, until recently, were considered to be outside the scope of nursing. These skills enable the nurse to systematically collect data about each body system, based on observation, measurement, palpation, auscultation and percussion. The interpretation of this data requires the nurse to draw on an expanded clinical knowledge base in order to differentiate the normal from the abnormal within the context of the individual concerned, their age and development, sex, ethnicity and culture (Estes 1998; Jarvis 2000). In addition, the advanced practitioner is able to identify and authorise further investigations such as laboratory tests.

The intended outcome of this total health assessment is primarily a nursing diagnosis. The North American Nursing Diagnosis Association (NANDA) defines this as a 'clinical judgement about individual, family or community responses to actual or potential health problems or life processes. Nursing diagnoses provide a basis for selection of nursing interventions to achieve outcomes for which the nurse is accountable', and help the nurse to identify those aspects of patient need that require the expertise of other health professionals (NANDA 1990; Carpenito 2002). Nursing diagnoses must be supported by clinical information that has been collated and summarised as a recognisable problem, the management of which is the legitimate remit of nursing (Sparks & Taylor 2001; Ackley & Ladwig 2002). Construction of the diagnosis takes place concurrently with the total health assessment as the advanced practitioner reviews information and assesses its significance in the light of possible explanations for the patient's condition (Burns 2002). As in medicine, working up a diagnosis is an inexact science in which the practitioner must consider and select from a range of possibilities (Seedhouse 1991).

The concept of nursing diagnoses has not been an explicit part of nursing practice in the UK. The nursing process was introduced as having four stages in which diagnosis was not mentioned. Nurses were taught that the intended outcome of assessment was the identification of the patient's problems and it was left to the individual practitioner to record these as they saw fit. However, in the 1970s, NANDA began to formally classify nursing diagnoses as part of legitimising nursing activities. As nursing became more independent there arose a need to develop a terminology that reflected its practice. Medical terminology was well-established and clearly understood and, therefore, American nurses sought to develop a similar system of communication. The work of NANDA has continued and nursing diagnoses are now included in Nurse Practice Acts, thus enshrining in law the nurse's professional right to diagnose within nursing.

Nurses in the UK are still working on issues of clarifying the nature and status of nursing. The recent work carried out by the Royal College of Nursing (RCN 2002: 1) highlights the lack of clarity about the nature of nursing and proposes that it be defined as 'the use of clinical judgement and the provision of care to promote, improve, maintain and recover health or, when death is inevitable, to die peacefully'. The specific characteristics of nursing are people's responses to and experiences of health, illness, frailty and disability; the promotion of health and healing; practice that is an intellectual, physical, emotional and moral activity in which the nurse works in partnership with patients and families and in collaboration with other professionals (RCN 2002).

The College goes on to argue that these proposed definitions are essential in response to the increased complexity of healthcare and changing social and professional roles. This is particularly pertinent to the introduction of advanced practice, the preparation for which equips practitioners not only to construct diagnoses within their own sphere of expertise but also, in certain circumstances, to make medical diagnoses and initiate appropriate treatment. Some medical colleagues will inevitably regard such activities negatively, questioning the legal right and expertise of non-doctors to perform such tasks and possibly seeing advanced practice as an encroachment on their professional turf. Moreover this perceived encroachment will not end with the performance of diagnosis. Proposals from the British Medical Association that nurses act as first-contact providers of healthcare in the community and care coordinators in acute settings will mean that more of what is currently considered day-to-day medical practice will become the province of suitably prepared nurses, leaving doctors free to look after patients with complex needs (BMA 2002).

Advanced and medical practitioners need to be clear about the nature and extent of each other's role if they are to collaborate effectively together. Inherent in the concept of collaboration are notions of equality and valuing another's expertise both of which are undermined by ill-defined work roles and suspicion (Hanson *et al.* 2000).

The problem-oriented/follow-up assessment

This type of assessment is directed towards the management of a specific health problem, such as Marcia's asthma, and requires the construction of a detailed database. In Marcia's case this will include information about the past history of her asthma, when it began, the severity and the identification of trigger factors such as foods or other substances. Physical measurements such as peak flow recordings will provide a baseline for the assessment of acute exacerbations of her asthma and the effectiveness of inhaler therapies. Construction of this database enables the advanced practitioner to spend time with Marcia, listening to her concerns and laying the foundation of a therapeutic relationship. The aim is to help Marcia lead as normal a life as possible by educating her about the nature of her condition and ways in which she can manage episodes of acute breathlessness and prevent long-term complications (Coakley 1999; Rees & Kanabar 2000). Spross *et al.* (2000) describe this activity as coaching and guiding the patient through a health/illness transition.

Transitions are characterised by change. They may mark a passage from one way of life to another, a change in status, circumstances or a combination of these elements. Coaching and guiding require the advanced practitioner to act as mentor and support by providing information in ways commensurate with the patient's ability to understand, helping that individual develop a positive approach to the management of their condition and ensuring that the individual is equipped to cope as their symptoms change. Coaching may involve formal teaching such as inhaler technique but is far more flexible, allowing time for the patient to rehearse situations known to provoke difficulties and explore different approaches to managing these. For example, at some point Marcia may wish to explore the benefits of non-allopathic therapies such as acupuncture, and the advanced practitioner can act as a sounding board, providing an opportunity to discuss the advantages and disadvantages of this therapy. Guiding refers to the ongoing assistance and supportive activities provided by the advanced practitioner in regular reviews of the patient's progress. It demands a high level of interpersonal competence that 'serves to bridge the differences between APNs and their clients and enables clients to share power and collaborate with APNs to develop a realistic plan of care' (Spross *et al.* 2000: 196). In this way the advanced practitioner is able to act as a resource without imposing solutions on the patient.

Conclusion

This chapter has examined some of the issues in the conduct of advanced health assessments and the different forms that these may take. Such assessments differ from those conducted by other nurses in that advanced practitioners are able to perform more detailed data collection that includes extensive physical examination and synthesise the information obtained with an expanded clinical knowledge base. However, if advanced assessments by nurses are to gain acceptance in the UK, then the interface between nursing and medicine must be further examined. Changes in both professions have called into question the type of practitioner society requires and expects each to be and identifies the need to redefine and legitimate new boundaries between the two.

? **Key questions for Chapter 8**

In your field of practice:

(1) To what extent does the definition of nursing proposed by the Royal College of Nursing reflect professional and advanced practice?
(2) In what ways does an expanded concept of health inform care currently provided in your workplace? Do you foresee any changes if advanced health assessments are performed?
(3) Is the nursing process appropriate and helpful for advanced practice?

References

Ackley, B. & Ladwig, G. (2002) *Nursing Diagnosis Handbook: A Guide to Planning Care*, 5th edn. St Louis: Mosby.

Bell, S. (1988) Becoming a political woman: the reconstruction and interpretation of experience through stories. In: *Gender and Discourse: The Power of Talk* (eds A.D. Todd & S. Fisher), pp. 97–124. Norwood, NJ: Ablex.

Benner, P. & Wrubel, J. (1989) *The Primacy of Caring: Stress and Coping in Health and Illness.* Menlo Park, CA: Addison-Wesley.

Benner, P., Tanner, C. & Chesla, C. (1996) *Expertise in Nursing Practice: Caring, Clinical Judgement and Ethics.* New York: Springer.

BMA (2002) *The Future Healthcare Workforce*, HPERU Discussion Paper 9. Available http://www.bma.org.uk

Burns, C. (2002) Advancing health assessment in pre and post registration nursing. Unpublished paper presented at an international seminar, University of Central England, April.

Carpenito, L.J. (2002) *Nursing Diagnosis: Application of Clinical Practice*, 9th edn. Philadelphia: Lippincott.

Coakley, L. (1999) *Health Education and Asthma.* Nursing Times Clinical Monograph No. 10. London: Nursing Times Books.

Cohen, S., Bailey, P.P., Begemann, C. & Mofett, K. (1998) Advanced physical assessment. In: *Advanced and Specialist Nursing Practice* (eds G. Castledine & P. McGee), pp. 93–118. Oxford: Blackwell Science.

Dunlop, M.J. (1986) Is a science of caring possible? *Journal of Advanced Nursing,* 11 (6): 661–70.

Dunphy, L. & Winland-Brown, J. (1998) The circle of caring: a transformative model of advanced practice nursing. *Clinical Excellence for Nurse Practitioners,* 2 (4): 241–7.

Estes, M.E. (1998) *Health Assessment and Physical Examination.* Albany: Delmar.

Hanson, C., Spross, J. & Carr, D. (2000) Collaboration. In: *Advanced Nursing Practice: An Integrative Approach* (eds A. Hamric, J. Spross & C. Hanson), pp. 315–48. Philadelphia: W.B. Saunders.

Jarvis, C. (2000) *Physical Examination and Health Assessment*, 3rd edn. Philadelphia: W.B. Saunders.

Leininger, M. (ed.) (1984) *Care: The Essence of Nursing and Health.* Detroit: Wayne State University Press.

Livo, N. and Rietz, S. (1986) *Storytelling: Process and Practice.* Littleton, CO: Libraries Unlimited, Inc.

McGee, P. (1998) *Models of Nursing in Action: A Pattern for Practical Care.* Cheltenham: Stanley Thornes.

Menzies. I. (1970) *The Functioning of Social Systems as a Defence Against Anxiety.* London: Tavistock Institute of Human Relations.

NANDA (1990) *Taxonomy of Nursing Diagnosis.* St Louis, NANDA.

RCN (2002) *Defining Nursing.* London: Royal College of Nursing.

Rees, J. & Kanabar, D. (2000) *ABC of Asthma*, 4th edn. London: BMJ Books.

Roper, N., Logan, W. & Tierney, A. (1990) *The Elements of Nursing*, 3rd edn. Edinburgh: Churchill Livingstone.

Roy, C. (1984) *Introduction to Nursing: An Adaptation Model*, 2nd edn. Englewood Cliffs, NJ: Prentice Hall.

Sandelowski, M. (1996) Truth/storytelling in nursing inquiry. In: *Truth in Nursing Inquiry* (eds J. Kikuchi, H. Simmons & D. Romyn), pp. 111–24. Thousand Oaks, CA: Sage.

Seedhouse, D. (1991) *Liberating Medicine.* Chichester: John Wiley.

Sparks, S. & Taylor, C. (2001) *Nursing Diagnosis Reference Manual,* 5th edn. Philadelphia: Springhouse Corp.

Spross, J., Clarke, E. & Beauregard, J. (2000) Expert coaching and guidance. In: *Advanced Nursing Practice: An Integrative Approach* (eds A. Hamric, J. Spross & C. Hanson), pp. 183–216. Philadelphia: W.B. Saunders.

Chapter 9

Reflecting on Mental Health Assessment and Advanced Nursing Practice

Dean Holyoake

'The goal of the advanced nurse practitioner's evolutionary process is to apply new knowledge, which is based on research, concepts and theories to the improvement of patient care.
(Sparacino 1992)

Imagine what a Martian would think of a nursing mental health assessment (MHA). What type of report would he write to send back home? How would he report that there are many different types, reasons for and ways to implement mental health assessments? As I reflect on what we mean by advanced nursing practice (ANP) and its relationship with mental health assessment it would be easy for me (and the Martian) to reproduce the hundreds of different types of scales that innumerable textbooks have already listed. But, I could also attempt to provide a more original exploration of what makes advanced mental health assessment different from what I call the primary or core types of mental health assessment. That is, I could attempt to comment on the way more and more mental health academics, practitioners and researchers are concerned with developing the process as an advancement of assessment protocol: the traditional 'use of self' and the advancement of the nurse–patient relationship as being representative of a total cultural 'advancement' with regard to the ideas we hold about assessment. This chapter does not intend to be a report back to Mars, but rather a reflection about the way mental health nursing has responded to and shaped the nature of assessment in practice with regard to promoting the relationship as the advanced nurse practitioner process of assessment.

Introduction

Assessment in mental health settings is not just a task that is implemented to 'get things under way'. Instead, it is a 'process' that connects all of the micro-level inter-actions that recur in the everyday interventions that mental health nurses have with their clients. Assessment is an ongoing process that is always informing and being informed by the nature and direction of treatment usually via the spoken word and the transference created by therapeutic relationships.

It is possible to explore assessment issues on at least two levels. First, there is the practical application of traditional and core assessment checklists that are closely allied to medicine and its positive roots. Examples here would include admission and initial interviews, ongoing observation (including observation checklists), the use of psychological assessments to rate depression, anxiety and so on to provide a 'baseline' from which to measure improvement and inform a diagnosis. This type of primary or core notion of assessment will always be the foundation of mental health nursing assessment, but there is a growing second opinion to accompany the traditional types of assessment and 'advance' the overall assessment in a number of ways. Many mental health nurses are beginning to take it upon themselves to improve the scales they use by analysing the nature of *relationship process* as a form of assessment as well as the outcome scores provided by the traditional assessment frameworks. In this way, their practice is boundary pushing in the spirit of advanced nursing practice. But I want to explore this more. The aims of this chapter are threefold and aim to trace the sequence of my reflection on the issue of assessment practice in mental health settings:

(1) To provide the reader with an introduction to the cultural issues associated with assessment in mental health settings
(2) To reflect on the traditional primary/core 'baseline'-type assessments and con-sider their benefits as well as their pitfalls
(3) To show how the impact of psychotherapeutic theory and practice is advancing mental health nursing assessments.

Culture, assessment and something called advanced nursing practice

> Advanced nursing practice has not been lost. (Castledine 1994)

Introducing the notion of advanced nursing practice

Even though the primary purpose of this chapter is to reflect on advanced nursing notions of assessment, it is important, and also a requirement, to say something about what advanced nursing practice is all about. With regard to the mental health arena, it can be argued that the impact of advanced nursing practice as a phenomenon was and is limited. This is not to be seen as a criticism of mental health nursing *per se*, but rather a statement that offers a reflection on the attempt during the 1990s of Anglo-American nursing academics to raise the profile of nursing. The suspicion of new titles, roles and objectives left no dents in most mental health units until the birth of the new nurse consultant role which, at both a political and practical consideration, has economic backing at most service contractual levels.

In mental health services today, there is a growing number of nurse consultants who are practising a role of the archetypal advanced nurse practitioner. Their experience, home grown-ness and pay have raised the status and respect they command within their specialities. Therefore, I am arguing that the development of advanced nursing practice as an expanded rather than extended role has not been in vain. The seeds that were sown are now beginning to germinate in readiness for harvest. A harvest of nurse consultants who have an objective of pushing boundaries, expanding practice and challenging longstanding psychiatric doctrine. Yet, it remains that the harvest festival may take some time. Figure 9.1 presents a synopsis of advanced nursing during the 1990s.

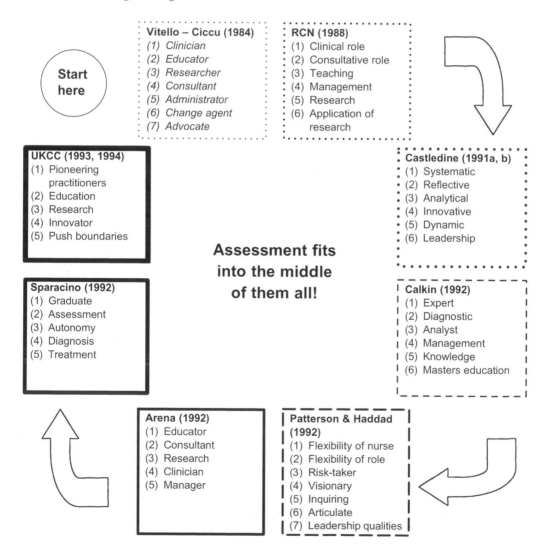

Fig. 9.1   The core facets of the ANP role (adapted from Holyoake 1998).

What is assessment?

Assessment is a question-generator in disguise and, like its half brother diagnosis, it occupies a particular space in what we as nurses do in our everyday practice. Issues related to intuition, experience and 'just knowing' the best course of treatment are all based upon what we 'observe' and the way we process observations to create more questions for testing. For this reason alone, assessment, as a core nursing task, has high-value symbolism.

How do mental health nurses actually use assessment in their everyday practice? What are the strategies that are employed either to maintain a unitary theoretical stance or to integrate ideas from different specialities? The simple answer to these questions point up the idea that most mental health nurses do not necessarily implement assessment strategies with the greatest degree of theoretical understanding. Instead, their major motivation will be to collect data about their patients so that they can at least begin an ongoing process of treatment and continued assessment, which is in some way informed, particularly in the community setting. It is assumed that the more experienced a nurse is, the more expert they are at making use of assessment data. In psychiatric culture there is a recognition that expert practice is founded on an ability of the expert nurse to get the most out of a situation. It reflects the notion that a better relationship with the patient enables a more informed and advanced type of assessment process. To be able to 'handle yourself' in assessment interviews is to demonstrate that you 'know your stuff' and can access good clinical judgement founded on years of experience. To be able to succinctly document observations and formulate modes of therapeutic intervention that can in turn be constantly assessed is the yardstick of core assessment. It is to this standard that most students and junior staff nurses aspire: to be able to assess their patients as having this or that problem within the first few hours. However unscientific and detrimental to the notion of expanding nursing practice in objective considerations, this type of intuition and its high-value symbolism belongs to a culture that has history (see Fig. 9.2).

To draw together this introductory first section, the important points relate to:

- the impact of cultural inferences (a specialisation relationship with medicine and psychiatry)
- the rise in appreciation for the constructionist world-view as opposed to a positivist one
- the high-value symbolism (in practice) of the expert practitioner.

These three points all have an impact on how assessment is implemented and accepted in mental health specialities. What, if anything, does this mean in practice? The following section reflects on this question.

Primary and core assessment in mental health nursing

> Posts suggest a defined economic response to the reality of individuals' aspirations.
> (Holyoake 1998)

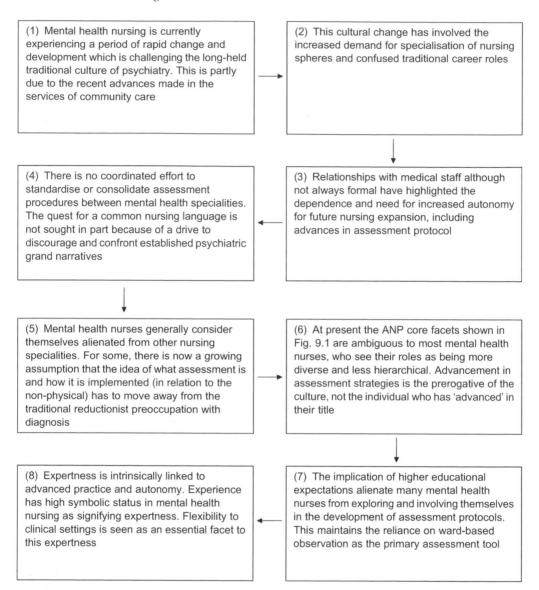

(1) Mental health nursing is currently experiencing a period of rapid change and development which is challenging the long-held traditional culture of psychiatry. This is partly due to the recent advances made in the services of community care

(2) This cultural change has involved the increased demand for specialisation of nursing spheres and confused traditional career roles

(4) There is no coordinated effort to standardise or consolidate assessment procedures between mental health specialities. The quest for a common nursing language is not sought in part because of a drive to discourage and confront established psychiatric grand narratives

(3) Relationships with medical staff although not always formal have highlighted the dependence and need for increased autonomy for future nursing expansion, including advances in assessment protocol

(5) Mental health nurses generally consider themselves alienated from other nursing specialities. For some, there is now a growing assumption that the idea of what assessment is and how it is implemented (in relation to the non-physical) has to move away from the traditional reductionist preoccupation with diagnosis

(6) At present the ANP core facets shown in Fig. 9.1 are ambiguous to most mental health nurses, who see their roles as being more diverse and less hierarchical. Advancement in assessment strategies is the prerogative of the culture, not the individual who has 'advanced' in their title

(8) Expertness is intrinsically linked to advanced practice and autonomy. Experience has high symbolic status in mental health nursing as signifying expertness. Flexibility to clinical settings is seen as an essential facet to this expertness

(7) The implication of higher educational expectations alienate many mental health nurses from exploring and involving themselves in the development of assessment protocols. This maintains the reliance on ward-based observation as the primary assessment tool

Fig. 9.2   Assessment, mental health nursing and a changing culture.

Models of assessment

As a short prelude, I want to note that during my research for this chapter it became evident that a great many nursing theorists and practitioners have written about assessment. Indeed, I counted at least 50 mainstream assessment protocols and packages that nurses are able to utilise in a number of settings. I also noticed that it is the tradition of every nursing textbook to have a chapter on assessment (including this one), all of which seem to repeat these said packages. Therefore, I have no regrets about not repeating this phenomenon. Instead, I want to continue my exploration into what the main core assessment procedures used by mental health nurses are in practice and, in particular, the way the therapeutic relationship is viewed as being fundamental to the overall process of assessment.

No matter what the impact of the culture, the necessity to assess and to at least begin to understand the nature of the patient's current condition is considered desirable, and even impossible to avoid, in most mental health settings. The acute unit with its emergency admissions, the elderly care units, forensic services, child and adolescent services, rehabilitation units, drug units and community settings all have core assessment which involves the interviewing of the patient, family members and liaising with other health professionals. The purpose of this section is to describe what happens in a lot of the settings. Figure 9.3 shows that there are many different types of core assessment frameworks available for use by mental health nurses. Some are more specialised than others, but in short, there is no limiting the number of possibilities for implementing ready-made assessment packages. Having said that, and as I will go on to explore in 'Travelling a journey', it is also the case that mental health nurses rely on a process of data collection that is inseparable from the fundamentals of initiating, in the first instance, a working relationship.

If we examine some of the core assessment possibilities shown in Fig. 9.3, it is possible to recognise not only the type of assessment but also the nature of the assessment process. For example, the admission interview and direct observation seem to speak for themselves, but are there any 'advances' that mental health nurses have used to adapt the nature of this type of assessment strategy? The use of self-monitoring by the client seems to be a novel and experimental type of strategy that has at its core an attempt to empower and involve the client in their own care. For example, when Sam had started to recover from a prolonged psychosis his key nurse suggested that he should contribute to his own notes. As a process this involved both Sam and his key nurse writing their own individual reflection on how Sam had presented during the day. The results showed that there was a high agreement and clarity in the key nurse's assessment of how Sam was presenting, thinking and feeling. The process allowed for daily focused discussion and a feeling for Sam that he was being listened to. This empathic journey also allowed for 'verbal self-reports' and a greater degree of therapeutic reflection. No longer was Sam expected to be passive and expecting of the fruitfulness of nursing assessment alone.

Likewise, Jenny during her sectioned admission to an acute psychiatric unit responded favourably to her key nurse's suggestion that she should keep a *diary* to

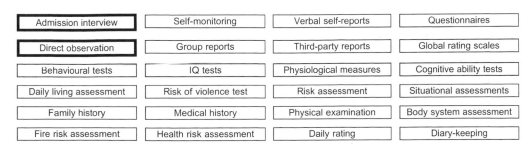

Fig. 9.3 Summary of the many different types of assessment frameworks.

help them both assess her progress. 'I'd never thought of keeping a diary, its seems so simple doesn't it, but I did. After about a couple of weeks we evaluated it and found that my insight was useful for us both. This story illustrates how, at a core level, attempting to promote the building of the therapeutic relationship led to the implementation of a simple assessment strategy. From here, her key nurse was able to involve Jenny in the development of *group reports* and *third-party reports* which entailed Jenny making a commitment to assessing her own motivation in group work and assessing how other people evaluated her behaviour: 'At first, it was strange, because it was like I was being invited in to talk about someone else, but it was really about myself ... like a sort of out of body experience.... People would say nice things to make me feel better, but eventually I was being exposed to the harsh truth about my self-harming.'

The idea of inclusion rather than exclusion is seemingly fundamental to the new wave of ideas that mental health nurses have about assessment. As Jenny quite rightly says, she was talking and writing about herself. She was being asked to document her own journey as an ongoing assessment. This process seems to contradict the old notions of the nurse filling in a tick-box form with the absence of a relationship and in some false belief that it was anything more than pseudo-scientific and therefore objective. Both Sam and Jenny become the credible authors and partners in their own health assessment. This is not to say that the pre-written risk assessments were not implemented, but as Jenny's key nurse noted: 'they were no longer the main assessment, in fact there are millions of these types of ready-made assessment, but there is only one Jenny's diary ...'.

The assessment interview and history-taking

In Fig. 9.3, it can be seen that both the *admission interview* (or in the case of community teams, the initial contact interview) and *direct observation* have been placed in heavy boxes. The reason for this is to emphasise them as the dominant processes by which mental health nurses glean assessment-type data about their patients. These two stand alone because they are the primary vehicles through which assessment is processed. Therefore, as the core methods of assessment they are worthy of further reflection. According to Bellack and Edlund (1992), the assessment interview has one of the following purposes: (1) to gain information, (2) to give information, or (3) to motivate. This is the basic function of the assessment interview usually carried out by a mental health nurse. An important point to recognise is that mental health nurses have a role in the admission for assessment of patients under the Mental Health Act 1983, that is any patient who is suffering from mental disorder of a nature or degree which warrants the detention of the patient in a hospital for assessment (DoH 1993). This was certainly the case for Jenny, as noted above.

The process of interviewing will usually go through a number of phases that include an *induction phase* (greeting, establishing rapport, gaining background data); a *working phase* that aims at fulfilling the stated purpose of the interview (gaining data regarding the nature of the patient's mental health needs); and finally the *termination phase* in which negotiation for further meetings and therapeutic work is contracted. The notion of process, that is the actual interaction between the nurse and the patient during the interview, remains the area that distinguishes the basic from the advanced in many ways. I will explore this in more detail in the following section, but for now it is important to point out that the Benner (1984) model seems aptly to reflect my point here. The notion that a more senior nurse is able to extract a greater detail of information, build better initial relationships and make intuitive judgements suggests that they are more expert due to having more exposure to this type of assessment task than that of a novice or advanced beginner. Although this should not strike us as being too unusual, it does start to suggest that assessment in mental health settings is related to the *use of self* as a tool rather than the simple completion of many of the established assessment tools. For example, a more experienced nurse will be able to provide more detail than a less experienced nurse even when they are both completing the same 'risk assessment tool' or 'family history'.

This notion of intuition and critical thinking is more about process, that is, how it is used, rather than the assessment tool itself. Therefore, the first point is that all types of 'basic assessment' (like the more unusual assessments discussed in the following section) can be further enhanced by the nurse who is operationalising them. So when a textbook carefully prescribes the verbal and non-verbal behaviours that nurses use to gather assessment data it suggests that all assessments in mental health can occur with some degree of regularity. Although this may be the case within a certain degree of continuum, I would suggest that 'basic' assessments are those that attempt just to 'get a result'. Something that enables a space in the patient's notes to be filled.

Observation (reporting and recording)

Some psychiatric conditions require a long stay in hospital: usually no less than four weeks and in many cases longer. This means that the nature of assessment is conditional on the needs of the client. It is becoming more recognised that if at all possible it is better to assess clients in their own homes. In the case of community teams this is possible for some types of referral, but for the most disturbed and acute illnesses, admission to hospital is another option. As part of the assessment process, a full medical and mental state examination should be followed by appropriate multidisciplinary discussion that enables the preparation of a treatment plan supported by further assessment. This assessment, usually via observation of the client, makes use of written documentation and can utilise observation checklists. One significant point I want to raise here (and will discuss in greater detail in the next section) is the role of the key nurse in *coordinating* a team of professionals who assess for different things in a number of different ways.

So far, I have noted that assessment is changing at both theoretical and practical levels. At the theoretical level, mental health nurses are becoming more concerned with the nature of their relationship as being just as important as the assessment tool outcomes. Also, there are hundreds of these assessment tools available. The use of the relationship as a dynamic of assessment harbours many of the humanistic aims of inclusion, empowerment and subjective-needs-led approach that sits comfortably within most psychiatric nursing cultures. This slow shift is a type of advancement in nursing in itself. Even though it is fragmented it can be seen in practice that nurses are taking more of a coordinating role and ensuring that multidisciplinary team assessment is grounded in the reality of the client. Now I want to continue my exploration by focusing on the way the therapeutic relationship reflects not only the basics of initial interviews and observations, but also advancements in the attitudes that more nurses now have about assessment.

Travelling a journey

> Assessment should be the first stage of any therapeutic intervention, it should not be seen as a 'one off'. (Marshall 1994: 351)

I have pointed out that owing to the relationship nature of the use of self as a tool, mental health nurses approach initial assessments (such as the admission interview) and the ongoing assessments of their patients (the daily observation and recording) with varying degrees of skill dependent upon their experience. When Janice, a clinical nurse specialist working with the elderly, told me she had implemented a number of scales to assess the toilet needs of her clients she was very careful to add: 'these scales enable us to be more evidence based ... but I know that the time I spend talking about the war is just as valuable in terms of assessing how someone is feeling'. Janice acknowledges that there is this 'process' element to the nature of assessment. So I asked her what are some of the more specialised and possibly 'advanced' modes of assessment that nurses are introducing. 'I think the scales allow us to justify treatment and make us feel as though the work we do is legitimate, but most nurses assess by *direct contact.'*

There is a desire by most mental health nurses to consider their patients holistically, contextually and as unique. This means a promotion of the use of self as the constant and consistent facet in any assessment process. At an epistemological level, this wish derives from a constructionist/constructivist world-view (with a humanist process level) as opposed to a reductionist, medical and positivist perspective, the latter being synonymous with psychiatry's attempt to medicalise itself and appear scientific in its everyday diagnosis and treatment of many illnesses that have no credible or indisputable known cause. Hence, when Janice said: 'I see my patients from day to day so I'm assessing all of the time ...', she is really speaking of mental health nurses pushing boundaries in the quality of the interactions they are now encountering with their clients and the care they take in ensuring a seamless evidence-based approach to teamwork. As noted by Tunmore (2000), skills in assessment are among the core skills of mental health nurses that the Sainsbury Centre report on the future roles and training of mental health staff identifies as core competences for these specialist staff (Table 9.1).

Paul, a specialist community mental health nurse working with drug users, told me: 'Assessment data is only as useful as the analysis and synthesis into meaningful patterns.... Every day, I have to identify and cluster cues, make activating hypotheses, and make clinical judgements.' This notion of clinical judgement begs the question, how do mental health nurses know what is the best type of assessment tool or approach for a particular patient? In the first place, they don't. Paul said: 'A relationship is started during the first interview, physical observations will be con-

Table 9.1   Core assessment skills (Tunmore 2000: 498).

- Appropriate values and attitudes
- Listening and questioning skills required to make accurate assessments of individual need
- Skill in conducting a collaborative needs-based assessment
- Ability to develop a treatment and care plan based on a thorough and comprehensive assessment of the client, family and social system
- Apply knowledge of the issues and skill in the assessment and management of the combined problem of drug/alcohol abuse and mental illness
- Apply knowledge and skill in risk assessment and the management of violence and aggression
- Apply knowledge of factors related to the development of 'chronic crises' and skill in assessment and management strategies

(Sainsbury Centre for Mental Health 1997)

ducted, medical history will be taken and initial observations will be recorded . . . it depends on the ability of the patient to give information. . . . I make a point of collecting assessment data from family members or carers.' To this point, the client can be said to have received all of the 'basic' or primary assessments. Now, depending on the nature of their illness, the speciality of the unit and the skill level of the nursing team will determine what, if any, types of further assessment they will receive during their assessment and treatment phases.

Figure 9.4 shows just some of the types of assessments, measures, examinations, tests and histories that mental health nurses implement. These are types of 'global assessment'. I spoke with Sandra, a charge nurse in a busy acute unit, who said: 'The emphasis is usually on the emotional, psychological and social lives of the patient . . . this is particularly important when you consider the implications of the Care Pro-

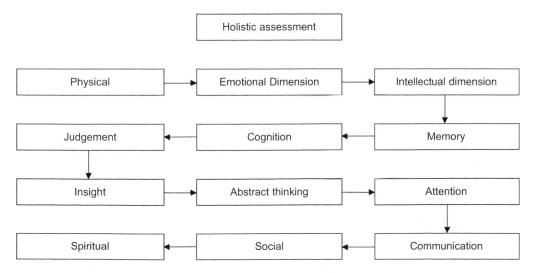

Fig. 9.4   An outline of 'global assessment' frameworks.

gramming Approach to care before discharge back home.' As both Sandra and I have alluded to, getting the most from any of these types of assessment tools and categories within holistic assessment frameworks is the responsibility of the people involved in the process. Therefore, advanced types of assessment occur when the nurse is aware that the *management of the process*, in particular the development of a *beneficial thera-peutic relationship*, is just as important for stimulating contextual data as the assessment tool itself. 'When I'd just started as a staff nurse I used to use checklist assessments and I was relieved when I'd managed to complete them . . . , but now I use the checklist to help me get into the shoes of the person I'm assessing, particularly if they are in a risk situation.' When Paul said this he indicated that understanding the reason why a particular assessment was useful has been at the core of understanding the difference between *primary* notions of assessment and *advanced* types of assessment. This point seems to be growing in recognition as more and more mental health nurses are working with specialised types of therapy and counselling frameworks.

Psychotherapeutic advancement – nursing assessment of the whole person

In comparison to the directives put forward by traditional assessment frameworks it is perhaps just as useful to consider the way mental health nursing has made use of psychotherapeutic assessments. These frameworks focus on the nature of the relationship and therefore are well-suited to the demands encountered by mental health nurses. The philosophical foundations of these *process-oriented assessments* are based on a similar world-view to that of more contemporary mental health. In addi-tion, many psychotherapeutic approaches attempt to provide new perspectives on the interface between the traditional diagnostic and the more intuitive approaches to psychotherapy (Clarkson 1992). This reflects my sentiments and the views of Janice, Paul and Sandra that diagnosis can be used to destructive or beneficial effect. In the words of Clarkson (1992: 55), 'this paradigm [psychotherapy] is intended to validate both a humanistic, person-orientated therapeutic relationship and to make the best possible use of information and patterns that have accrued from our historical and scientific predecessors in the field of psychotherapy and psychiatry'. Figure 9.5 gives an overview of the guiding principles by which mental health nurses are viewing assessment of 'the whole person'.

Mental health nurses like Paul, Sandra and Janice are beginning to re-evaluate traditional forms of medical assessment because they are concerned to reflect the principles shown in Fig. 9.5. The work of Barker (1990, 1996) gives evidence to suggest that mental health nurses are now tending to adopt a more holistic approach to assessment with a more credible understanding of ethical and moral dimensions to their practice. This concern for the 'more unconventional' is illustrated by Stroll (1979), who offers a useful guide for spiritual assessment and, as noted by Narayanasamy (1994), includes an appraisal about concepts of God, sources of strength and tradi-tional spiritual practices. Advances in assessment no longer seem to be primarily about what criteria should be included, but rather, how these criteria can help to sustain an ongoing therapeutic relationship that reflects the live relationship of the client and nurse. Clarkson (1992) sums it up by stating: 'An over-reliance on diagnosis can create false certainties if used in a restrictive, insensitive way leading to cookbook

Assessment results are not secret or written in pseudo-medical jargon. 'Anything that is not worth saying in front of the patient is not worth saying at all' (Berne, cited in Steiner 1974: 6)	'Everything diagnosed [and assessed] psychiatrically unless clearly organic in origin, is a form of alienation' (Steiner 1974: 16)	The centrality of the relationship is swinging the 'historical pendulum away from diagnosis, which is seen to be contrary to and destructive of the creative, growthful encounter between two people in psychotherapy' (Clarkson 1992: 56)
Psychiatric diagnosis and assessment have often been used in a reductionist and pseudo-medical controlling manner. Mental health nurses in their everyday practice are opting to use more humanistic and socio-cultural assessment instead	Research suggests that warmth, acceptance, respect, empathy and genuiness are associated with positive outcomes of psychotherapy (Lambert 1986)	'For many people in psychotherapy the establishment of a significant relationship with a client or patient is of the greatest importance' (Rogers 1986: 171)

Fig. 9.5   Guiding principles underpinning holistic mental health nursing practice.

treatment planning, an emphasis on sameness, an avoidance of valuing cultural or temperamental idiosyncrasies and an adherence to techniques or labels.'

Mental health nurses in their isolated pockets are now beginning to assert themselves more than ever in an attempt to advance useful assessment protocols in their own specialisms, the main issue being a quest for assessment, diagnosis and treatment that enables the patient to be unique, individual and involved. It is no longer acceptable to apply standard types of assessment checklist and claim that an assessment 'has been done'. Advanced assessments are about travelling a journey with the patient from initial assessment to discharge that is not steered by false and premature certainty that some assessment formats provide. This journey involves exploring a better understanding of the frequency, intensity, nature and duration of assessment processes that are client-led as opposed to what Paul described as 'an out-of-date beginning to the nursing process ... just something that we have to do'.

Conclusion

The notion of nursing assessment is well-documented. Most good nursing textbooks will have lists and taxonomies of the categories and types of question to ask. These same textbooks will also demonstrate the importance of the 'how to do' interviewing by spending considerable amounts of time highlighting issues to do with verbal and non-verbal communication and so on. But like the Martian writing home, I have tried to provide a reflection on what seems to be a consolidation of practice in mental health settings today. The three main points I have raised during this reflection have a direct relationship to those things that I have not done. First, I have not provided pages and pages of references to the hundreds of already tested assessment packages that have been developed. I have not done this partly owing to the fact that others have done a much better job than I am capable of and partly owing to the idea that my reflection has been more concerned with process than with outcome. Perhaps this in itself can be seed as an 'advanced nursing academia'. The second point relates to the idea of process and the 'use of self' as having a direct impact on the nature of the assessment period for both client and nurse. Although it might have been useful to explore issues related to strategic developments at an organisational or even national level, I have been content to restrict myself to the more personal. Accounts lent to me by the nurse leaders I spoke to regarding the nature of their assessments in practice in which they remembered being novice and now take it upon themselves to advance practice as experts, helped me to reflect on point three, which concerns the impact that psychotherapeutic theory and practice have had on mental health settings. Probably more than any other influence, the use of psychotherapeutic approaches to practice has sunk into the bones of mental health nursing culture. Assessment is not just the start of a therapeutic journey, but the guide and map that helps both the client and nurse along the undiscovered path.

? **Key questions for Chapter 9**

In your field of practice:

(1)   What are the characteristics of professional and advanced health assessments?
(2)   To what extent is the therapeutic use of self an essential element of advanced practice?
(3)   In what ways can the advanced practitioner actively enable patients to take an active role in assessment as described in this chapter?

References

Arena, D. & Page, N. (1992) The imposter phenomenon in the CNS role. *Image Journal of Nursing Scholarship*, 24: 121–5.

Barker, P. (1996) *Assessment in Psychiatric and Mental Health Nursing: In Search of the Whole Person.* Cheltenham: Stanley Thornes.

Barker, P. (1990) The philosophy of psychiatric nursing. *Nursing Standard*, 5 (12): 28–33.

Bellack, J. & Edlund, B. (1992) *Nursing Assessment and Diagnosis*, 2nd edn. Boston: Jones & Bartlett.

Benner, P. (1984) *From Novice to Expert: Excellence and Power in Clinical Nursing Practice.* Menlo Park, CA: Addison-Wesley.

Calkin, J. (1984) A model for advanced nursing practice. *Journal of Nursing Administration*, January: 24–30.

Castledine, G. (1991a) The advanced practitioner: part one. *Nursing Standard*, 5 (43): 34–6.

Castledine, G. (1991b) The advanced nurse practitioner: part two. *Nursing Standard*, 5, (44): 33–5.

Castledine, G. (1994) UKCC's standards for education and practice. *British Journal of Nursing*, 3 (5): 233–4.

Clarkson, P. (1992) *Transactional Analysis Psychotherapy: An Integrated Approach.* London: Rout-ledge.

DoH (1993) *Mental Health Act 1983: Code of Practice Revision and attached further proposed amend-ments.* London: DoH.

Holyoake, D. (1998) Advanced nursing practice in a culture of mental health nursing. In: *Per-spectives of Advanced Nursing Practice* (eds P. Thorbrook & G. Rolfe), pp. 177–98. Oxford: Butterworth-Heinemann.

Lambert, J.J. (1986) Implications of psychotherapy outcome research for eclectic psychotherapy. In: *Handbook of Eclectic Psychotherapy* (ed. J. Norcross), pp. 436–62. New York: Brunner/Mazel.

Marshall, S. (1994) Cognitive behavioural therapy. In: *Lyttle's Mental Health and Disorder*, 2nd edn (eds T. Thompson & P. Mathias), pp. 345–60. London: Baillière-Tindall.

Narayanasamy, A. (1994) *Spiritual Care and Mental Health Competence.* In: *Lyttle's Mental Health and Disorder*, 2nd edn (eds T. Thompson & P. Mathias), pp. 367–84. London: Baillière-Tindall.

Patterson, C. & Hadad, B. (1992) The advanced nurse practitioner: common attributes. *Canadian Journal of Nursing Administration*, 5 (4): 18–20.

RCN (1988) *Specialities in Nursing.* London: RCN.

Rogers, C. (1986) *Client-centered Therapy.* London: Constable.

Sainsbury Centre for Mental Health (1997) *Pulling Together: The Future Roles and Training of Mental Health Staff.* London: Sainsbury Centre for Mental Health.

Sparacino, P. (1992) Advanced practice: the clinical nurse specialist. *Nurse Practitioner*, 5 (4): 2–4.

Steiner, C.M. (1974) *Radical Therapist/Rough Times Collective: The Radical Therapist.* Harmonds-worth: Penguin.

Stroll, R.G. (1979) Guidelines for spiritual assessment. *American Journal of Nursing*, 79: 1574–7.

Tunmore, R. (2000) Practitioner assessment skills. In: *Lyttle's Mental Health and Disorder*, 3rd edn (eds T. Thompson & P. Mathias), pp. 482–504. London: Baillière-Tindall.

UKCC (1993) *The Council's Proposed Standards for Post-Registration Education and Practice.* London: UKCC.

UKCC (1994) *The Future of Professional Practice – The Council's Standards for Education and Practice following Registration.* London: UKCC.

Vitello-Ciccu, J. (1984) Excellence in critical care: educating the clinical specialist. *Critical Care Quarterly*, 21: 1–2.

Chapter 10

Advanced Practice and Health Promotion

Ann Close

Introduction

In performing advanced health assessments the advanced practitioner demonstrates a commitment to an expanded and holistic concept of health. In this context neither society nor professionals define health. It is not an ideal, unattainable state but a changing state of being experienced by the individual in response to events both within and outside that person. Health is more than the absence of disease and it is possible for the two to coexist within the individual. Thus a person with diabetes may describe herself as 'well for me'. This expanded idea of health has created opportunities for advanced practitioners to engage with individuals and populations in a wide variety of settings to promote an understanding of factors that affect health and how these may be managed. Individuals cannot take responsibility for every aspect of their health but there is, nevertheless, much that they can do to reduce the risk of serious illness or to minimise the potential complications of particular diseases or conditions.

This chapter begins by considering current ideas about the nature of health. Included here is a discussion of health beliefs. Consideration of an individual's beliefs about health can reveal that person's values and priorities as well as the influence of family, friends and culture. This in turn will indicate how much control the individual is able to exert over their personal circumstances. Those who believe that they can affect their own health are more likely to be able to take more positive action than those who do not. Beliefs about health are a fundamental in health promotion and this chapter moves on to present a discussion of this topic with particular reference to developing personal skills and risk assessment. The final section of the chapter examines the potential for health promotion within the advanced practice role at both national and local levels.

The nature of health

Health is a value judgement that individuals make based on their goals, beliefs and aspirations and shaped by their social and cultural experiences. Health can be seen as having the following components:

- *Physical health* that is concerned with the physical functioning of the body, including certain aspects of fitness such as strength and stamina, characteristics such as body size and shape, susceptibility to infection and ability to recuperate.
- *Mental health* refers to the ability to learn, to grow from experience, to think clearly and coherently and the ability to solve problems.
- *Social health* that includes the ability to make and maintain satisfying interpersonal relationships, respond appropriately in various social situations and fulfil a role in society.
- *Emotional health* refers to the ability to express emotions such as joy, fear and grief appropriately in terms of both manner and place, cope with stress and deal with other emotional reactions and tensions.
- *Spiritual health* includes the feelings of unity with others, principles of behaviour and personal values and, for some people, religious beliefs and practices (Coutts & Hardy 1985; Ewles & Simnett 1986).

Ewles and Simnett (1986) argue that, whilst these different aspects of health are useful in demonstrating the complexity of health, they should not be seen as separate concepts. Instead they should be seen as interrelated and interdependent, thus providing a holistic view of an individual's health and wellness or well-being.

Health is not just the absence of disease and illness. It is also about an improved quality of life. Several authors refer to health as being about maximising potential or adding value to life. Seedhouse (1986, 1991) sees health as working towards attaining potential. Health is not only how the individual is now but also what they may become in the future, in both positive and negative terms. Tones (1996) takes the view that health is linked to a socially and economically productive life. Doyal and Gough

(1991) support this, arguing that health is the ability to participate in life. Overall these views of health suggest that health is a dynamic, lifelong process aimed at achieving potential and participating in society. A range of factors constantly influences this process provoking responses and adaptations (Smith, 1992; Benzeval *et al.* 1997; Jones 1997). For example, lifestyle is currently regarded as having a profound influence on health. An unhealthy lifestyle, or in some cases modern/western life, is now regarded as a principal contributor to sickness and disease, precipitating a range of initiatives aimed at informing members of the public about the perils of living as they do and the risks they incur (Peterson & Lupton 1996).

This notion of educating people about lifestyle is predicated upon the concept of the person as a rational, calculating individual capable of making informed choices when provided with the necessary information, and the idea that making such choices is both a right and a responsibility. In reality the ability to make any kind of choice is constantly modified by numerous factors, such as sex, class, personal circumstances, level of education and intelligence, that are outside the individual's control – a situation that can have negative consequences that include blaming the victim for failing to change when provided with information (Seedhouse 1988; Jenson & Mooney 1990).

Allied to the notion of lifestyle is a change in the notion of the body (Peterson & Lupton 1996: 23). The body is more than a matter of staying healthy or free from disease. The body has become a major part of the presentation of the self to the world, a 'project to be worked on'. The body can be altered or even partially reconstructed to fit prevailing fashions/individuals' desires. Working on the body is a constant chore requiring education to help the individual make suitable choices and invest personal effort to avoid backsliding. The ideal body is slim, toned, has a flat stomach, is free of blemishes, looks good in designer labels but is more than just a fashion statement. It is also an expression of the individual striving to maintain health and demonstrate personal responsibility. Advanced practitioners must recognise that the emphasis on lifestyle, and in particular the body, is very much a western construct and that each culture promotes its own views of how the body should be and be seen (Helman 2000).

Health beliefs and behaviours

An understanding of the factors that influence health beliefs and subsequent health-related behaviours will help the advanced practitioner understand what makes individuals behave as they do in order to plan more effective health promotion strategies. There is a range of theories and models that attempt to explain the link between health beliefs and health-related behaviour. Three are presented here as examples to show the complex nature of human behaviour in relation to health.

Socio-cognitive theory

Socio-cognitive theory is important in helping to understand and predict behaviour and to identify methods in which behaviour can be modified and changed. It is particularly relevant to health promotion. The basis of the theory is that a person's expectations, beliefs, self-perceptions, goals and intentions give shape and direction to behaviour. In addition, biological and personal factors such as sex, ethnicity, temperament and genetic make up also have an influence on behaviour. Bandura (1977, 1986) suggests that behaviour can be predicted and explained by the following concepts:

- *Response consequences* that act as incentives for taking action or changing behaviour, such as improved health, increased comfort, prevention of illness. The degree to which the individual values these incentives will influence the extent to which they are likely to follow a course of action and change behaviour.
- *Outcome expectancy*, that is the extent to which the individual believes that the action will result in the desired outcome;.
- *Efficacy expectancy*, which refers to how confident the individual feels in undertaking, achieving and maintaining the new behaviour or action.
- *Vicarious learning* or learning by observing others, which allows an individual to develop a new idea without actually performing the behaviour. It is important as it enables learning without trial and error and can avoid mistakes. Individuals are more likely to model behaviour they observe displayed by those they identify with, such as role models they see as similar to themselves.
- *Self-efficacy*, which is a type of self-reflection that affects behaviour. Individuals develop perceptions about their own abilities which subsequently guide their behaviour by influencing what they will try to achieve and how much effort they put into doing this. Self-efficacy develops as a result of a person's previous experiences of achievement, from observing the successes and failures of others, listening to the views of others and the physiological status, including feelings of anxiety or elation at the time. Comparison with others also determines self-efficacy.

An understanding of socio-cognitive theories will assist advanced practitioners in planning health promotion to meet individuals' needs. Someone with low self-efficacy will need short-term, achievable goals that they value, actions or learning which is broken down into easy stages, opportunities to observe others in the same situation who have achieved success, and frequent positive feedback.

Health locus of control

The health locus of control was derived from social learning theory by Rotter (1954) and is concerned with the extent to which individuals believe that their health is controlled by what they do (internal factors) or by events outside their personal control (external factors). Wallston and Wallston (1981) further developed the locus of control unidimensional continuum that measures the degree to which people believe their health is or is not determined by their own behaviour. They suggest that beliefs about health control fall into three categories:

- I – *internal*, which is the extent to which one believes that internal factors are responsible for health and illness

- P – *powerful* others is the belief that one's health is determined by powerful others such as healthcare professionals or family members
- C – *chance*, which measures the extent to which one believes that health and illness are a matter of chance.

Various studies have found that social and demographic factors such as economic status, age, sex, family background and occupation affect the locus of control; for example, people of a low socio-economic status tend to believe that health is more likely a result of fate or chance (Calnan 1988). Health locus of control theory is important for advanced practitioners as it highlights the importance that having a sense of control plays in behavioural change. If people believe that they can take action to solve a problem or influence their health in a positive way they are more inclined to do so and feel more committed to the course of action agreed.

The health belief model

The health belief model was originally developed in the 1950s and 1960s by three social psychologists: Hochbaum, Kegels and Rosenstock (McCormack Brown 1998). It attempts to explain what motivates people to engage in activities aimed at preventing and avoiding disease and what encourages them to seek healthcare services. The health belief model suggests that an individual's motivation to seek healthcare is determined by several perceptions that the individual holds:

- Their level of susceptibility – the extent to which the individual feels at risk of developing the disease or condition.
- The severity of the condition – that concerns the individual's beliefs about how serious the condition is and the effects it might have on their personal and working life.
- The benefits – the extent to which the individual believes the intervention will be effective in preventing the condition or reducing its seriousness.
- The barriers – the extent to which the individual feels the barriers he must confront, such as inconvenience, expense and pain, are worth it.

The health beliefs model recognises that there are additional modifying factors such as age, sex, ethnicity and socio-economic factors. In addition, there are cues to action that make the individual aware of potential health risks. These include TV and newspaper stories, mass media campaigns, illness in family or friends (Rosenstock 1974). The model can help advanced practitioners to understand how their patients perceive themselves in relation to an actual or potential health problem and plan the health promotion strategies accordingly.

There is a great deal of overlap between the different theories and models of health beliefs and behaviours. However, they do highlight the many factors that are believed to influence people's health beliefs and motivate them in different situations. Individuals are more likely to engage in positive health behaviours if they have an incentive, they believe the action will have the result they want and they are capable of achieving it. An understanding of these theories is essential in assisting advanced practitioners to plan health promotion activities and motivate patients.

What is health promotion?

Health promotion is a term used to encompass many activities. The Ottawa Charter (WHO 1986) identifies five components of health promotion:

- *Healthy public policies.* This refers to the need to have wider public health, social and economic policies that include legislation and regulations designed to protect people's health. Examples include, tobacco control and regulations on smoking in public places; wearing of seat belts and crash helmets, and drug control measures.
- *Creating supportive environments.* This involves creating conditions that will enhance health and well-being through protecting the natural and the 'man-made' environment. It includes the green policies for cutting global and atmospheric pollution, the provision of better public transport and leisure and recreation services. Links have been made between healthy public policy and the supportive environment. In 1990 it was claimed that, 'the main aim of Healthy Public Policy was to create supportive environments which would make health choices possible or easier for the citizens and enable them to lead a healthy life' (WHO 1990). This message was reinforced in the Sundsvall declaration in 1991 (WHO 1991).
- *Strengthening community action.* This refers to the importance of supporting local residents and groups in the community to improve their health by setting priorities and plans and taking action locally. It aims to facilitate cooperation and empower communities, including workplaces, to take more responsibility for their health by actively participating in making healthy choices. Local workplaces in the community can also be included.
- *Developing personal skills.* This involves personal and social development through health education. According to Sidell (1997), health education is 'a form of communication which aims to give people the knowledge and skills needed to make choices about their health'. This requires:
  - awareness raising, bringing an issue to the attention of the individual and influencing their agenda
  - helping the individual to acquire knowledge and skills about the health issue
  - helping that person clarify their values and change their attitudes and beliefs
  - helping them link their attitudes to behaviour changes
  - helping them focus on goals that are important to them.
  Health education is an important component of health promotion as it supports the other elements. Awareness-raising, the development of knowledge and skills, appropriate attitudes and communication are essential for developing effective policies and for involving and empowering communities to participate and create conditions where individuals can be more healthy and choose a more healthy lifestyle.
- *Reorienting health services.* This recognises that health services must move beyond providing curative care to adopt a more health promotion role and recognise that

many other services such as housing, economics, transport, leisure and recreation have an influence on health.

Healthy alliances

Healthy alliances encourage partnership between individuals and organisations in order to promote health. Adams (1992) defines such alliances as 'a partnership for health gain that goes beyond health care and attempts collectively to change the social and environmental circumstances that affect health.' To be successful, Douglas (1998) suggests organisations in any alliance should have a shared purpose, mutual trust and sufficient needs on the part of the participants to make joint work worthwhile. He also recognises there are a number of significant challenges for organisations in healthy alliances including the need for them to:

- Identify and control the real costs of inter-agency working
- Maintain clear and coherent leadership across the organisations
- Develop seamlessness so that there is continuity for patients
- Manage the joint priorities that emerge
- Handle the impact on workers from each organisation
- Measure and evaluate the results of collaboration
- Review and modify the alliance as necessary.

Alliances can be established at international, national, regional and local levels, and the Department of Health publication *Working Together for Better Health* (DoH 1993) provides guidelines on how to set up and maintain an alliance.

There is an increasing requirement to work in collaborative partnerships in the NHS to improve the health of individuals and reduce inequalities. The NHS Plan (DoH 2000) acknowledges that the NHS cannot tackle health inequalities alone and states that a key strategic role for health authorities is to develop new partnerships between health and local services to strengthen the links between health, education, employment and other causes of inequality. These include new public health groups across NHS regional and government offices to enable the regeneration of regions and a Healthy Communities Collaborative to spread best practice in conjunction with the Health Development Agency.

Risk reduction and risk management

According to Beck (1992), we are living in a 'risk society'. This is particularly so in healthcare, which is not just concerned with cure and treatment but also interested in identifying, managing and monitoring risk factors which may indicate future illness. The process of managing risks in the health promotion context is no different from risk management in other situations. There are five elements in risk management. First, actual and potential risks must be identified. This is done by collecting evidence through research, audit and experience. For example, over decades, smoking has been identified as the leading single cause of avoidable ill health and contributes to such things as stroke, heart disease, vascular disease, low birth weight and prenatal mortality. Second, consciousness of the risk must be raised at different levels, for example with the government, which can then develop healthy public policies with health, education and local authorities, so that they can introduce local strategies and health promotion campaigns; and with individuals so that they are aware of the risks and can consider taking preventative action. Third, there must be an assessment of the risk. This can be done at different levels and in different ways:

- *Population screening* or epidemiological surveys that attempt to identify the distribution and levels of disease, deaths, disabilities and other disorders as well as healthy growth, development, behavioural and other factors which determine health across populations. Such surveys will influence the health improvement plans (HIMPs) of health economies.
- *Personal health check-ups* that include the wide range of check-ups and screening that is available throughout life, including postnatal screening, cervical screening, mammography, blood and urine checks and more specific targeted genetic testing.
- *Detailed individual assessments* that may be undertaken if a potential problem is identified through general screening. For example, a blood screening test may show a raised cholesterol level and this may be followed by a detailed assessment of all the risk factors related to heart disease.
- *Managing or reducing the risk*, which involves planning and taking actions that will reduce or manage the risk; for example, introducing legislation to reduce accidents such as traffic calming measures and speed restrictions or, at a more personal level, changing diet to reduce fat and cholesterol intake to reduce the risk of heart disease.
- *Evaluation* that involves reviewing the actions taken to determine the effect on the health of the population or the individual.

Models of health promotion

A variety of health promotion models emerged in the 1980s and 1990s (Tannahill 1985; Ryder & Campbell 1988; Beattie 1991; Ewles & Simnett 1992; Tones 1996). These are useful to advanced practitioners in that they form a framework showing how different components of health promotion interact. They provide the opportunity for practitioners to examine their practice and challenge underlying assumptions. There is no one, perfect, comprehensive model for every occasion, which means that models can be used eclectically to guide the practice of health promotion (Kemm & Close 1995). Two of the models of health promotion are described below.

The Tannahill model

The Tannahill model (Tannahill 1985) describes three overlapping components of health promotion: disease prevention, health education and tertiary protection. There are three types of disease prevention:

- Primary prevention or health promotion that attempts to prevent the onset of disease, for example vaccination programmes, lifestyle changes or preventing road accidents by making roads safer.
- Secondary prevention or early detection of disease before it causes symptoms, such as breast and cervical screening and action to reduce disease progression, for example drugs such as those used to lower cholesterol.
- Tertiary prevention that prevents recurrence of disease or prevents it from causing complications such as modifying lifestyle following heart attack or foot care for diabetic patients.

Health education may be preventative, for example, giving dietary advice or working with groups in the community or workplace to create positive health education to build up life skills and demand changes to the environment. Health protection is aimed at preventing ill health, for example through the fluoridation of water or campaigning for protective legislation regarding seat belt usage, alcohol consumption and driving, and health and safety at work (Table 10.1).

The Ewles and Simnett model

The Ewles and Simnett model (1992) describes five approaches that offer different ways of thinking about health promotion. Although health professionals from different backgrounds may favour a particular approach, the approaches are not necessarily discrete and advanced practitioners may find using aspects of more than one approach helpful. The dominant approach used by advanced practitioners should be the one they feel most comfortable with and which meets patients' needs. The five approaches are:

- *Medical approach*, in other words a medical intervention is required to prevent or improve ill health. This approach relies on patients complying with the prescribed preventative measures. For example, in patients who are obese the aim would be freedom from diseases related to obesity such as diabetes, heart disease and stroke, by encouraging them to reduce weight through diet and exercise.
- *Behaviour change approach*, the aim of which is to change people's attitude and behaviour as defined by the health professional. It relies on people adopting healthier lifestyles. For example, in patients who are obese this would involve persuading and educating them about following a sensible diet, eating the right foods and encouraging them to take more exercise. Ewles and Simnett (1986) acknowledge that this approach is based on three assumptions: that the healthcare professional, as the expert, knows best; that professionals can impose their values on the patient, and that an individual is genuinely free to choose a healthy lifestyle.
- *Educational approach*, which is aimed at giving knowledge to others and ensuring that they understand health issues. The approach is based on the premise that if individuals have knowledge and understanding they can make informed decisions and choices. For example, patients are given information about different types of diet and exercise regime and then supported in learning how to incorporate these in their daily lives. In this approach the health professional's values or views have

Table 10.1   Using the Tannahill model of health promotion in relation to chronic obstructive pulmonary disease (COPD).

Dimension of health promotion	Example
Primary prevention	Advice on effects of smoking and passive smoking Exploring attitudes in relation to smoking General health advice
Secondary prevention	As above plus: Advice and support on smoking cessation Advice and help with nicotine replacement interventions Advice on avoiding triggers to asthma attacks Early assessment and diagnosis Lung function tests to detect specific type of problem, e.g. spirometry Appropriate preventative drug therapy, e.g. bronchodilators
Tertiary prevention	As above plus: Managing infections Flu vaccination Advice on weight reduction Avoidance of activities which invoke breathlessness Advice on COPD prevention Effective management of COPD
Health education	Giving advice on the effect of smoking Advice on smoking cessation Building life skills with individuals that will help them resist peer pressure and demand changes to the environment such as smoke-free environments Promotion of non-smoking as the norm
Health protection	Tobacco control measures, restricting advertising, restrictions on age for smoking and smoking in some public places Health warnings on cigarette packs and adverts Restrictions on emissions of atmospheric pollutants Restrictions of using noxious substances at work environments Smoke-free policies in workplaces

less influence as patients are encouraged to make choices, although the professional determines what knowledge is given and in what way.

- *Client-centred approach* is one in which individuals set the agenda and then make their own decisions and choices according to their own interests and not those imposed by healthcare professionals. For example, diet and/or exercise issues are considered only if patients identify what, if anything, about these subjects they want to know. This is often difficult for people, however, as they frequently rely on health professionals to tell them what they do not know.

- *Social change approach* is one that aims to instigate political or social action to change the environment to facilitate the choice of a healthier lifestyle, for example through healthy eating choices, exercise programmes in schools, workplaces and hospitals. The idea is that the healthier option should also be the easiest choice to make.

Opportunities for health promotion in advanced nursing practice

The models and theories in this chapter provide a framework for advanced practitioners to promote health by influencing policy-makers and other influential groups at national and local levels, commissioners of healthcare, communities, individuals and groups and health professionals. The potential contribution of the advanced practitioner to each of these is discussed below.

Influencing policy-makers at national level

In order to influence policy-makers, advanced practitioners should be able to identify the degree of risk to the population of a particular health problem or disease and the factors that contribute to its development. Assessing risk will require the advanced practitioner to work with public health colleagues and policy-makers to critically appraise and synthesise the evidence from relevant research, evaluation studies, audits and professional opinion in order to construct a picture of the national situation. An examination of skin cancer provides an illustration of how this level of influence may work.

Case study: Skin cancer

Skin cancer is primarily due to sunburn and is caused by the harmful effects of UV radiation. The ozone layer in the atmosphere protects us from the harmful effects of some types of UV radiation. Skin cancer is the second most common cancer nationally, and its incidence is rising, with 40 000 new cases per year and around 2000 deaths. Nine out of ten of these cancers are non-melanomas, usually occurring in the over 50s and outdoor workers, and are due to cumulative exposure to the sun. The remaining 10% are malignant melanomas usually occurring in 20–35 year olds and linked to occasional exposure to periods of intense burning sunlight. These are the most serious and fatal skin cancers. National governments have begun to take action to reduce the depletion in the ozone layer, by restricting the use of chlorofluorocarbons in refrigerators, foam blowing agents and propellants in sprays. Local councils provide a service for disposing of old refrigerators. Weather forecasters also contribute by using the solar UV Index on a scale of 1–20 to advise viewers on the risk of sunburn. Although the NHS Plan (DoH 2000) has cancer as a major target, skin cancer does not feature as high on the agenda as some other cancers. Sun awareness campaigns are not as prominent as those for cervical and breast screening. Advanced practitioners may be in a position to influence developments for skin cancer through their professional associations and groups.

Influencing commissioners of healthcare

Primary care trusts have the responsibility of commissioning care to meet the health needs of their local populations. This responsibility is outlined in the Health Improvement Plan and agreed in the Service and Financial Framework (SaFF) agreements between the trust and each of its providers. The agreements set out the level and standard of service to be provided and the costs. The NHS Plan (DoH 2000) promotes the role of nurses and midwives in taking a lead in the way local health services are organised and run. Advanced practitioners are in a prime position to influence the commissioners on what is needed to meet the needs of the patients in relation to their speciality.

Case study continued

Most skin cancers are preventable if the right action is taken or they can be detected early and curative treatment instigated because people know what to look for. Although commissioners have a good overview of the health of the local population, they do not have the same detailed understanding and knowledge as the advanced practitioner about the condition or the group of patients, and their focus is often on care and treatment rather than prevention and early detection. Advanced practitioners must, therefore, be involved in developing both the Health Improvement Plan for their local health economies and the SaFFs to raise commissioners' awareness of the importance of including health promotion strategies and campaigns for skin cancer.

Influencing communities

People in specific communities, including schools and workplaces, are often keen to improve their health but do not always have sufficient knowledge or skills to do this. Although the health of such communities may not be the direct responsibility of advanced practitioners, they may still play a significant role in getting things started or in providing support and advice.

Case study continued

Following a national advertising campaign a local community group has been made aware of the risk of skin cancer and wants to take some local action. The aim of running a campaign locally is to provide basic information, increase awareness, motivate people to take action and show them how to carry that action through. In working in this way the advanced practitioner should consider the following:

- Involving others such as schools, local authority, employers, occupational health departments, health promotion services, local businesses and local media who may be able to provide help, support and sponsorship
- Focusing events to happen at a particular time, such as a sun awareness week, to get maximum publicity

- Promoting general awareness in the community by advertising and news articles in the local press, radio and TV and posters in public buildings such as libraries and health centres
- Undertaking visits to specific groups such as nurseries, schools and workplaces to create interest and involvement appropriate to the age, culture and ethnicity of different groups through talks, competitions, quizzes, and using role models such as pop stars, sports heroes
- Seeking sponsorship from pharmaceutical companies or local businesses to provide gift packs with materials to promote sun protection such as sun hats, sun screen, cartoon pictures showing when the sun is at its hottest and when to avoid it
- Taking part in health checks and fairs that offer opportunities for the public to obtain more information on early detection and also to consult a health professional over their individual concerns
- Encouraging members of the community to develop seating in shaded areas in parks and public gardens.

Influencing individuals and groups

Advanced practitioners can influence groups and individuals by developing programmes to raise awareness, assisting them in acquiring new knowledge and behaviours, and focusing on what is important to them. It is important the patients are involved and consulted to determine what they want. Developing programmes involves conducting an advanced health assessment that includes physical and mental health, values, attitudes, lifestyle and spiritual beliefs as well as details of social circumstances that indicate the extent to which others may influence an individual's behaviour. Existing knowledge and sources of health information will also be included to determine how much the individual knows, in this case, about skin cancer, the effects of the sun, methods of sun protection and how that person accesses information, for example through health professionals, popular magazines, friends or others.

This assessment will help the advanced practitioner to plan, deliver and evaluate an education programme, setting aims and objectives that focus on the individual's learning needs and taking into account what can be achieved in the time available. The education plan will include strategies and resources to help the patient learn. Planning and delivering such a programme requires effective communication that facilitates the exploration of feelings and attitudes, provision of information and the practice of skills. The advanced practitioner needs to develop a repertoire of education strategies to meet the needs of different groups. For example, children learn best through play and by imitation and they tend to have a short attention span. Adults learn best in familiar, non-threatening environments and in response to a perceived need. Older people tend to require a slower pace of learning with repeat demonstrations and procedures that are explained carefully and slowly. People like different media to support learning and the younger population in particular like electronic formats. Whatever materials are chosen, they should be reviewed for their suitability for use with a specific group or individual and should be employed only if they enhance learning in some way. There are many types of written, audiovisual and interactive

Table 10.2 Health promotion and skin cancer prevention: education programme for families to reduce risks of skin cancer.
Target population: mother aged 30 years with children aged 5 and 8 years old

Learning objective The mother will be able to:	Content	Strategies and learning materials	Evaluation
Explain what skin cancer is	Malignant melanoma Non-malignant melanomas: • Basal cell carcinoma • Squamous cell carcinoma	Verbal explanation with pictures of different types of cancer	Are they able to explain what skin cancer is?
Explain the factors that contribute to skin cancer and identify if the family is at high risk	Sunbathing in short intense bursts, e.g. weekends and holidays (risk of malignant melanoma) Prolonged exposure (risk of other skin cancers) Effects of ozone layer Age Family history Fair skin	Verbal explanation Explore family history and habits and link to potential risks Reinforce with leaflet to take home	Are they able to identify the factors that contribute to skin cancer? Can they relate this to their own lifestyle and changes they might need to make?
Explain how to avoid the contributory factors and protect family members	Protective clothing and benefits of natural cotton Sunglasses which conform to European standards Sunscreen (Factor 15 and above; Factor 30 for children) Correct application of sunscreen Avoid tanning beds Avoid sun at hottest times Information from weather forecasters Use of shade	Verbal explanation Demonstrate application of sunscreen to ensure adequate cover Provide with giftpack for children Leaflet as above Cartoon leaflet for children	Can they identify what protective measures are available? Can they identify the hours and times of year when the sun is at its hottest? Are they able to demonstrate how to apply sunscreen effectively?
Explain how to carry out skin checks	Frequency of skin checks What to look for Where to look Record of checks Contact GP for anything unusual .	Demonstrate checking process Supervise patient Questions and answers Provide leaflet 'Skin checking'	Are they able to demonstrate how to check their own skin? Can they explain what they are looking for? Can they record this accurately?

materials which have different uses, advantages and disadvantages of which are outlined by Kemm and Close (1995). The overall effectiveness of the programme should be evaluated to determine the extent to which learning and changes of behaviour have occurred and whether the programme was cost effective (Table 10.2).

Influencing health professionals

It is not easy for advanced practitioners to tackle health promotion alone and they need to get the support of other health professionals. This might involve sharing knowledge with and influencing colleagues and helping them develop the necessary skills and attitudes to deliver health education programmes. Examples of how this may be done are set out in Table 10.3.

Table 10.3   Influencing health professionals to participate in skin cancer prevention.

Health professional	Action
Clinical leaders, e.g. nursing and medical directors	Develop and promote organisational strategies relating to skin cancer prevention Encourage clinical staff to promote sun awareness
Managers	Ensure organisational policies and strategies are implemented Focus resources on specific activities
Ward managers/health centre managers	Display information about skin cancer and sun awareness
Multidisciplinary teams	Give information and materials on sun awareness to patients and families
Chief executive and human resources director	Ensure all staff are given information on sun awareness

Conclusion

Advanced practitioners carry out a number of interrelated functions. They are experts in whatever is their field of practice and draw on advanced knowledge and highly specialised technical and clinical interventions. They are able to exercise leadership at different levels which they can use to improve standards and quality and develop best practice as well as acting as a resource and support to others. They can also take a lead in shaping services to meet patients' needs. They use their knowledge and expertise to help identify the training and development needs of all members of the multidisciplinary team and they are in a position to conduct and apply research in practice to improve patient care. All of these skills are essential in health promotion. The advanced practitioner is in a prime position to influence the development and implementation of health promotion policies, motivate communities and health professionals to participate, and encourage them to develop the knowledge and skills required to create effective health-promoting practices.

> **?** **Key questions for Chapter 10**
>
> In your field of practice:
>
> (1) How could the advanced practitioner identify the health beliefs of and influences upon, the client population?
> (2) What strategies would be most appropriate for the advanced practitioner in promoting health and how might these be evaluated?
> (3) In what ways could the advanced practitioner influence the commissioners of health care?

References

Adams, L. (1992) cited in Powell, M., *Healthy Alliances: Report to the Health Gain Standing Committee*. London: Office for Public Management.

Bandura, A. (1977) *A Social Learning Theory*. Englewood Cliffs, NJ: Prentice Hall.

Bandura, A. (1986) *Social Foundations of Thought and Action*. Englewood Cliffs, NJ: Prentice Hall.

Beattie, A. (1991) Knowledge and control in health promotion: a test case for social theory and social policy. In: *Sociology of the Health Service* (eds J. Gabe, M. Calnan & M. Bury), pp. 162–202. London: Routledge.

Beck, U. (1992) *Risk Society: Towards a New Modernity*. London: Sage.

Benzeval, M., Judge, K. & Whitehead, M. (1997) Tackling inequalities in health: extracts from the Summary. In: *Debates and Dilemmas in Promoting Health* (eds M. Sidell *et al.*). Basingstoke: Macmillan.

Calnan, M. (1988) The health locus of control: an empirical test. *Health Promotion*, 2: 323–30.

Coutts, L.C. & Hardy, L.K. (1985), *Teaching for Health – The Nurse as Health Educator*. Edinburgh: Churchill Livingstone.

DoH (1993) *Working Together for Better Health: Health of the Nation*. London: DoH.

DoH (2000) *The NHS Plan: A Plan for Investment, A plan for Reform*. London: DoH.

Douglas, R. (1998) A framework for healthy alliances. In: *Alliances in Health Promotion: Theory and Practice* (ed. A. Scriven). Basingstoke: Macmillan.

Doyal, L. & Gough, I. (1991) *Towards a Theory of Human Needs*. Basingstoke: Macmillan.

Ewles L. & Simnett, I. (1986) *Promoting Health: A Practical Guide to Health Education*. Chichester: John Wiley.

Ewles L. & Simnett, I. (1992) *Promoting Health*, 2nd edn. London: Scutari Press.

Helman, C. (2000) *Culture, Health and Illness*, 4th edn. Oxford: Butterworth-Heinemann.

Jenson, U. & Mooney, G. (1990) *Changing Values in Medical and Health Care Decision Making*. Chichester: John Wiley.

Jones, L. (1997) Behavioural and environmental influences on health. In: *Promoting Health: Knowledge and Practice* (eds J. Katz *et al.*). Basingstoke: Macmillan.

Kemm, J. & Close, A. (1995) *Health Promotion: Theory and Practice*. Basingstoke: Macmillan.

McCormack Brown, K. (1998) Health behaviour change: theories and models. University of Florida Community and Faculty Health Online Service.
Available at http://www.med.usf.edu/~kmbrown/hlth_beh_

Peterson, A. & Lupton, D. (1996) *The New Public Health: Health and Self in the Age of Risk*. London: Sage.

Rosenstock, I.M. (1974) The health belief model and preventive health behaviour. In: *The Health Belief Model and Personal Health Behaviour* (ed. M. Becker). Thorofare, NJ: Charles Slack.

Rotter, J.B. (1954). *Social Learning and Clinical Psychology*. Englewood Cliffs, NJ: Prentice Hall.

Ryder, J. & Campbell, L. (1988) *Balancing Acts in Personal, Social and Health Education*. London: Routledge.

Seedhouse, D. (1986). *Health: The Foundations for Achievement*. Chichester: John Wiley.

Seedhouse, D. (1991) *Liberating Medicine*. Chichester: John Wiley.

Seedhouse, D. (1988) *Ethics: The Heart of Health Care*. Chichester: John Wiley.

Sidell, M. (1997) Educating for health. In: *Promoting Health: Knowledge and Practice* (eds J. Katz & A. Peberdy), pp. 155–72. Basingstoke: Macmillan.

Smith, A. (1992) Setting a strategy for health. *British Medical Journal*, 304: 376–8.

Tannahill, A. (1985) What is health promotion? *Health Education Journal*, 44: 167–8.

Tones, K. (1996) The anatomy and ideology of health promotion: empowerment in context. In: *Health Promotion: Professional Perspectives* (eds A. Scriven *et al.*). Basingstoke: Macmillan.

Wallston, K. & Wallston, B. (1981) Health locus of control scales. In: *Research with the Locus of Control Construct* vol. 1 (ed. H. Lefcourt). New York: Academic Press.

WHO (1986) *Ottawa Charter for Health Promotion: An International Conference on Health Promotion*, November 17–21. Copenhagen: WHO.

WHO (1990) *Investment in Health*. Brochure prepared for the International Conference on Health Promotion, 17–19 December.

WHO (1991) *Sundsvall Statement on Supportive Environments for Health*, 9–15 June. Stockholm: WHO.

Chapter 11

Cultural Competence and Advanced Practice

Paula McGee

Introduction

Culture is an important part of who we are and how we interact with the world. It provides learned ways of thinking and feeling that significantly affect the development of our attitudes, values and beliefs. Culture is shared with others and provides a particular way of being in and experiencing the world. It is a type of 'mental software' that shapes both groups of people and their individual members (Hofstede 1994: 4). The importance of culture in nursing care has been gradually established during the past twenty years. Current ideas about the nature and reasons for this change of values are linked to three factors: a better understanding of the relationships between culture, health, illness, treatment and care; the impact of the legislation on human rights; current health and social care policy. Actively incorporating culture into care is regarded as a dimension of the moral work of nursing in helping people to make sense of their illness or disability in ways that are meaningful to them and in doing so helping them to accept and enjoy their life (Mendyka 2000). Failure to take culture into account devalues others' experiences and beliefs and can contribute to the perpetuation of health inequalities.

This chapter focuses on cultural competence, a particular theoretical approach to the incorporation of culture into nursing care. Within this theoretical approach there are several competing theories and three are examined here. The chapter closes with a discussion of cultural competence in relation to two aspects of advanced practice. First, theoretical ideas are examined in relation to patient care and, in particular, nursing assessment. Second, cultural competence is examined in relation to the provision of clinical and professional leadership.

The concept of competence

Nursing is in many ways driven by the concept of competence in that practitioners are required to demonstrate their ability to practise safely both for entry to the Register and in order to further their careers. Given the emphasis on competence it is surprising to find that there is no agreed definition, no clear agreement on what it is. First, competence may be regarded as a continuum, as the antithesis of incompetence. In pre-registration education the student is required to progress towards a set standard by demonstrating competence in assessing, planning, implementing and evaluating care. Once qualified, practitioners are required to maintain their competence and improve on it. Allied to this idea of a continuum is the notion of competence as observable behaviour based on behavioural taxonomies. Students are assessed in the performance of skills and are seen as progressing through a series of stages from novice to expert. There is an element of measurement in this type of competence and some conflation of competence with performance (Lilyman 1998).

A third interpretation of competence is that of critical thinking: the ability to question and analyse using reflective and scholarly skills, both during and after a clinical event, to inform clinical reasoning and decision-making (Brechin *et al.* 2000). This type of competence is a complex web of attributes, knowledge and skills that acknowledges the complexity of modern healthcare and suggests that there is more than one way of practising competently (Lilyman 1998). This notion of competence is evident in recent debates surrounding post-registration practice. The United Kingdom Central Council (UKCC 1994) initially proposed three forms of post-registration practice that eventually became levels of practice (UKCC 1999). The Department of Health also identified three levels: professional, specialist and consultant (DoH 1999). If there are levels of nursing practice then it makes sense to argue that there are also levels of competence. Notions of competence as a continuum may be helpful in determining fitness for registration, but beyond that, professional competence may be better viewed as a continuous striving to improve, to achieve the next level.

Cultural competence and advanced practice

The notion of competence as an evolving state is central to all theoretical ideas about cultural competence. It arises from the recognition that learning our own culture takes a lifetime of experience that begins in infancy. So much of what we learn is taken for granted and we are never called upon to question it until we meet someone culturally different from ourselves. It follows that learning about the values and beliefs of other cultures, and the ways in which these inform practices relating to healthcare and the management of illness, will also take time because information will be obtained from diverse sources, pieced together gradually and must then be checked to ensure accuracy. Adaptations in nursing practice occur alongside an unfolding under-standing of patients' ways of experiencing the world.

Theoretical ideas about cultural competence are well established, but it is only recently that that these have featured in the discourse about advanced practice. Demographic changes that have occurred as a result of migration have presented a series of challenges to healthcare systems rooted in western European traditions. During the 1990s the USA has experienced rapid increases in population in minority ethnic groups, particularly those of Hispanic origins. It is estimated that by 2010 some states will no longer have a single dominant culture and that the level of diversity across the country will require health professionals to interact with members of almost every culture in the world (Echols 1998; Salimbene 1999). The UK has experienced similar change although not on the same scale. Minority ethnic groups still comprise a small proportion of the population as a whole but they are not evenly dispersed geographically. Thus health professionals have to be able to meet diverse local needs. Advanced practitioners are ideally placed to provide leadership in identifying local needs and acting as role models, demonstrating ways of adapting practice or intro-ducing new ventures.

Numerous research studies in the UK have demonstrated that people who are members of minority ethnic groups suffer health inequalities (see, for example, Evers *et al.* 1988; NAHA 1988; Balarajan and Raleigh 1995; Kelleher & Hillier 1996; Nazroo 1997; McGee 2000; Papadopoulos 2002). Reasons for this include, inappropriate ser-vices and stereotypical assumptions (Evers *et al.* 1988; Ahmad 2000), poor commu-nication (Cortis 1998), variations between groups in terms of morbidity and mortality (Nazroo 1997; Erens *et al.* 2001), and lack of knowledge among health professionals (McGee 2000). Racism is also evident both in the behaviour of staff towards patients, patients' treatment of staff and the ways in which staff interact with one another (Beishon *et al.* 1995; Ahmad & Atkin 1996; Darr 1998; McGee 2000; Notter & Klem 2001). The outcomes of the inquiry into the death of Stephen Lawrence and the later introduction of the Human Rights Act required all public services to address 'insti-tutional racism' which the inquiry's report defined as 'the collective failure of an organisation to provide an appropriate service to people because of their colour, culture or ethnic origin. It can be detected in processes, attitudes and behaviour which amount to discrimination through unwitting prejudice, ignorance, thoughtlessness and racist stereotyping which disadvantage minority ethnic people' (Home Office 1999: para. 6.34).

Cultural competence is, therefore, required of all health professionals. The recent National Service Frameworks (for example, that for older adults (DoH 2001)) make it clear that, to meet each standard, services must take account of the needs of local members of minority ethnic groups. There are additional issues at stake here. If members of minority groups feel that services are inappropriate to their needs, they are unlikely to make use of them except as a last resort. Consequently, when they do seek help they are likely to be more ill and cost more to treat. This is certainly the case with other marginalised groups such as the homeless whose health and life expec-tancy are far worse than the mainstream population and who experience high levels of stigma and social exclusion. Studies of nurse practitioners in the UK have demonstrated that suitably qualified and experienced nurses, with good interpersonal skills, can build effective therapeutic relationships with homeless people. Such nurses can act as first-contact professionals, providing treatment and care for patients who may have multiple and complex needs. The nurses were pivotal in developing and maintaining collaborative working with other professionals and agencies on the streets. They could also act as advocates for homeless people needing help from mainstream health services (McGee 1999). Advanced practitioners working with minority ethnic groups could perform a similar role, making services more accessible, sensitive and responsive to local needs.

Approaches to cultural competence

There are a number of theories about the provision of culturally competent nursing care. Three are discussed below.

Campinha-Bacote's theory

Campinha-Bacote (1994a) defines cultural competence as a process of ongoing development in which the nurse continuously strives towards working effectively within the cultural context of an individual or community (Fig. 11.1).

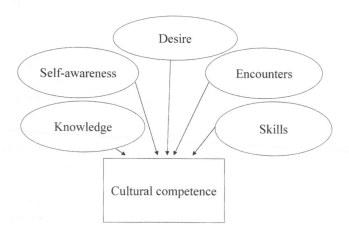

Fig. 11.1   Campinha-Bacote's theory of cultural competence.

- *Cultural awareness* is a deliberate, conscious process of examining the self that is strongly linked with *cultural desire*, the motivation to learn about diversity and develop the skills required for culturally-competent practice. Cultural awareness and desire requires nurses to develop an understanding of cultural differences and prejudice within their own lives. Interactional style is a particular concern because it arises from cultural values and beliefs. Nurses need to recognise the potential for misunderstanding, and even conflict, that may arise when they and their patients use very different styles (Campinha-Bacote 1994b, 1996). Nurses must examine the ways in which their own negative attitudes and prejudices affect their interactions with people from other cultures and 'strive toward a culturally-liberated inter-acting style' in which differences are seen positively as part of 'a shared learning experience' with the patient (Campinha-Bacote 1994a, p. 9). The object is to become culturally responsive by 'incorporating the individual's beliefs, lifeways and practices into a mutually acceptable treatment plan' (p. 11).

- *Cultural knowledge* is a process through which the nurse, or organisation learns about 'the various world views of cultures' by drawing on transcultural nursing, transcultural psychiatry, anthropology and medical anthropology (Campinha-Bacote 1994a: 12). Central to this is knowledge of the ways in which culture influences beliefs about health and the causation of illness. Included here are culture-bound illnesses[1] such as 'mal ojo' (evil eye) (Campinha-Bacote 1994a, b, 1996). The nurse must acquire an understanding of the specific health problems and needs of members of particular cultures by developing 'the skill necessary to obtain cultural knowledge directly from the client' in order to prevent stereotyping members of specific groups and to ensure that judgements made about treatment and care are accurate (Campinha-Bacote 1994a: 19).

- *Cultural skill* requires the application of cultural knowledge to patient care. The main skill area identified is that of patient assessment for which the nurse can select from a range of established, cultural assessment tools. Applying such tools requires the acquisition of a culturally appropriate interactional style that develops, over time, through stages in which the nurse passes from the avoidance of cultural questions in assessment to feeling confident in initiating conversation on this subject (Campinha-Bacote 1994a). Competence is dependent on the skills of listening to the patient's views, explaining one's own views, acknowledging similarities and differences in these, making professional recommendations and negotiating a treatment plan – factors that could also form part of an organisation's plan for cultural competence (Campinha-Bacote 1988, 1994a, 1995, 1996).

- *Cultural encounter* is a process of directly engaging in cross-cultural care situations. These serve both to reinforce learning and to challenge inappropriate attitudes or inaccurate knowledge as a basis for 'a sound framework in developing culturally relevant care interventions' (Campinha-Bacote 1994a: 30; 1994b). There is a fairly extensive body of literature that supports the need for encounters particularly through immersion in a new/foreign culture. St Clair and McKenry (1999) for example, researched students before and after clinical electives outside the USA using Likert-type scales and other tools. Students showed significant changes in behavioural and attitudinal factors following the experience of being *the other* when compared with their peers, who stayed behind.

Lipson and Steiger's theory

Lipson and Steiger (1996) provide an alternative view of cultural competence by basing their ideas on the concept of self-care, which, they argue, is a universal

---

[1] Culture-bound illness refers to conditions that are recognised only within specific cultures and which have little or no meaning elsewhere. An UK example is the notion of 'catching a chill'.

dimension of culture. In all cultures, individuals are expected to perform certain things for themselves and to call on family or social networks when help is needed. Self-care in this context refers to 'health related activities in which individuals, families or communities take part on a regular basis' and is distinguished somewhat tenuously from self help which is defined as a group approach to problems (Lipson & Steiger 1996: 13). Self-care is based on the assumption that people are responsible for their own health regardless of social or class boundaries. The main components of self-care are health promotion and maintenance, disease prevention, detection and management. Cultural competence depends on the nurse's ability to develop the *cultural perspective*. This has three elements: the self, the other and the context (Fig. 11.2).

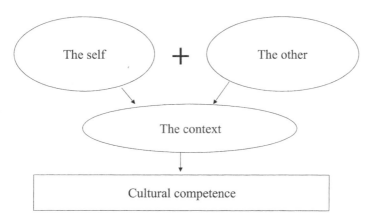

Fig. 11.2 Lipson and Steiger's theory of cultural competence.

The element of *the self* requires that the nurse examine personal values and beliefs, culture and other factors that may affect cross-cultural communication such as the lack of a shared language between patient and professional. Lipson and Steiger (1996) provide guidance on working with interpreters and draw attention to other factors, such as time orientation, that may affect communication. Competence in cross-cultural communication can develop through four stages, from unconscious incompetence in which the nurse misinterprets the patient's meaning but is unaware of this, to conscious competence in which effective communication takes place without conscious effort (Fig. 11.3).

The element of *the other* requires the nurse to learn about the patient, family and community with regard to ideas about health, illness and self-care. This involves developing knowledge of specific cultural groups and the circumstances in which

• Unconscious incompetence = unaware of the cultural dimensions of the situation • Conscious incompetence = aware of cultural dimensions but chooses to ignore them/displays prejudice • Conscious competence = understands what is required but has to make a conscious effort • Unconscious competence = understands what is required and can act without conscious effort

Fig. 11.3 Levels of competence.

they live as a basis for conducting cultural assessments that should include religion, language, health beliefs and food. In contrast to Campinha-Bacote (1994a), Lipson and Steiger (1996) go on to outline the incorporation of assessment data into the planning and implementation of care. Competence is linked to the application of knowledge and skill within the framework of the nursing process.

Finally, the nurse must consider *the context* in which this application of knowledge is taking place. This idea of context is the least well-developed aspect of Lipson and Steiger's (1996) ideas, but they argue that the nurse must have an understanding of the ways in which society treats members of black and other minority ethnic groups and the factors that may deter individuals from seeking help.

McGee's theory

McGee (2000) proposes an approach to cultural competence that draws on these perspectives but which also incorporates her own research, the work of Benner *et al.* (1996) and that of Ramsden (1995) who argued the importance of cultural safety in care. In this theory, cultural competence is a continuous process of *learning, performing and reflecting* that enables individual practitioners and healthcare teams to provide safe and meaningful care (Fig. 11.4).

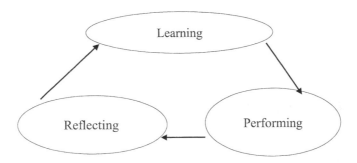

Fig. 11.4 Cultural competence is a continuous process.

The focus on *learning* requires nurses to clearly identify their patient groups (Fig. 11.5a). This means moving beyond descriptive statistics such as admission figures to develop good quality, detailed and meaningful data. For example, a trust finds that 20% of admissions in the last year were people who originated in the Indian sub-continent. A more detailed database would reveal which areas they originated from, how long they have been settled in the UK, languages spoken, religion, values, specific health problems and so on. Such information may, of itself, reveal particular health needs and shortcomings in current services.

Learning also requires practitioners to focus on themselves, to develop an awareness of themselves as cultural beings with their own values, beliefs and attitudes and how these may affect the nurse–patient relationship (Fig. 11.5a). Inevitably, developing this awareness will include identifying one's own strongly held views or even prejudices towards those whose way of life is very different. Sands and Hale (1987)

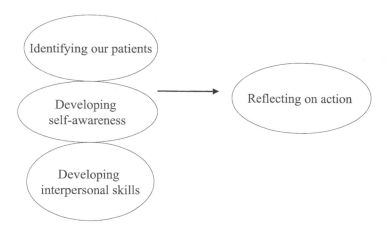

Fig. 11.5(a)   McGee's theory of cultural competence: learning and reflecting.

have described an approach to this subject by asking nurses to consider how they deal with patients of whom they in some way disapprove and to develop strategies to minimise the effect of that disapproval on the delivery of care.

Finally, learning requires developments in interpersonal skills (Fig. 11.5a). These include the ability to recognise and adapt to diverse styles of interaction and observe differing cultural mores associated with polite behaviour, for example in greetings, using eye contact, non-verbal signals and issues surrounding gender. Included here is the recognition that nurses and patients may not share a common language and the need to ensure effective communication, for example by working with interpreters.

The performance of nursing care provides opportunities for nurses to apply their learning and add to their understanding of cultural issues in care. *Reflection* informs and refines learning. Competence increases gradually, based on theoretical and experiential knowledge that is checked and tested through caring for patients (Figs 11.5a, b). Even when mistakes occur, the process of reflection enables practitioners to reconceptualise their understanding of an event and clarify the learning required to

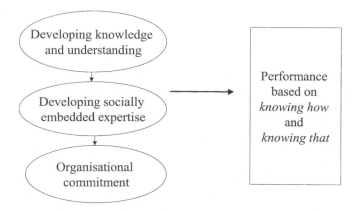

Fig. 11.5(b)   McGee's theory of cultural competence: learning and performing.

prevent a recurrence. However, individual competence cannot be enough because episodes of patient care are usually shared among members of a team, particularly in hospital settings. Membership of the team provides nurses with opportunities to develop *socially embedded expertise* by sharing knowledge through informal conversation or demonstration. Such sharing exposes individual team members to multiple perspectives that help 'to limit tunnel vision and snap judgements' and provides 'powerful strategies for maximising the clinical knowledge of a group' (Benner *et al.* 1996: 205). In this way competence moves from being an individual attribute to one that is team-based so that patients receive a similar standard of care irrespective of who is on duty.

The principle of socially embedded expertise can be extended to the whole organisation (Fig. 11.5b). For culturally competent services to become a reality there must be *organisational commitment* to change that is made evident in mission statements, policies, procedures and, most importantly, financial allocations (Malone 1993; McGee 2000). A culturally competent organisation demonstrates respect for its clients and staff by upholding cultural values and beliefs.

This overview of theories about cultural competence demonstrates a number of shared themes. First, cultural competence requires professionals to focus on themselves both as cultural beings and, in the case of McGee (2000), as representatives of organisational culture. Second, the ability to facilitate effective communication between members of different cultures is critical. Third, professionals need a constantly expanding theoretical and experiential knowledge base about their client groups. Finally, the social context of care, particularly that of health services, is influential. The implications of these for two aspects of advanced practice are discussed below.

Culturally competent nursing assessment and advanced practice

One of the key elements of advanced practice is the ability to perform advanced health assessments based on a holistic and systematic approach to the individual that includes collecting physical data, a full health history, data from diagnostic tests and other information including culture. The object is to use the assessment to formulate a nursing diagnosis that informs the planning and delivery of nursing interventions (Estes 1998; Andrews 2000). Addressing the cultural dimension of the assessment involves the 'systematic appraisal of an individual's beliefs, values and practices' for the purpose of 'providing culturally-competent healthcare' (Andrews 2000: 46). This appraisal requires the advanced practitioner to understand the cultural values of the patient with regard to health and healthcare (Fig. 11.6). There are two schools of thought on how this should be done. The first states that general assessment frameworks can be used to generate sufficient information alongside other types of data (Rooda 1992). Whilst this may appear to be a very sensible approach, an examination of general assessment frameworks indicates that culture is usually a minor consideration. For example, one of the most commonly used frameworks for nursing assessment used in the UK is based on the work of Roper *et al.* (1990). This framework does not address cultural issues in any depth. McGee (2000) found that it did not

• Customs and rituals	• Culture-specific syndromes
• Language and communication styles	• Ways of expressing illness, pain etc.
• Family and social relationships	• Values, beliefs and practices related to health
• Conceptualisations of the body, health and illness	and healthcare
	• Variations in morbidity and mortality

Fig. 11.6 Cultural dimensions of advanced health assessment.

encourage nurses to focus on cultural issues and was of limited value in this aspect of patient assessment.

The second view is that the assessment of cultural issues should be a separate activity and be based on a specialised framework (Leininger 1995; Andrews & Boyle 1999). There are numerous frameworks to choose from but they share the same fundamental weakness in that they are all lengthy and complex. Indeed, De Santis (1994) has estimated that some would require up to two years of intensive fieldwork and are, therefore, impractical. Moreover, the separate assessment of culture does not help professionals to integrate the information obtained with that concerning the patient's state of health.

Alongside consideration of assessment tools are issues concerning the collection and interpretation of data across different cultures. In any nurse–patient interaction there can be several cultures present. First, the nurse and the patient each have their own personal cultures that define their values, beliefs and ways of life. Second, the nurse is a member of a professional culture with its own norms, values and expectations. Finally, the organisation within which the nurse and patient are brought together also has a culture that affects the ways in which care is delivered. Thus the nurse is a member of several cultures each of which may require different ways of interacting with and regarding the patient. In such circumstances, achieving an accurate understanding of the patient's views and problems becomes a difficult and complex task requiring the nurse to check that information is correctly interpreted. At the very least the advanced practitioner needs to have experience of working with a range of different cultural groups, preferably those represented in the locality, and have the opportunity to check the interpretation of information with other members of the patient's culture. Simple, intuitive interpretation is not valid and failure to assess correctly can lead to misdiagnosis and inappropriate treatment (Paniagua 1994).

This discussion demonstrates that culturally competent nursing assessment is still evolving and there is, so far, no one approach that is entirely satisfactory. This situation presents a number of opportunities for advanced practitioners. First, they need to work towards achieving cultural competence in their own practice by embarking on a process of becoming culturally self-aware. Alongside this they will need to use their scholarly skills to evaluate approaches to culturally competent assessment and to develop a knowledge base about local cultures. This may include a formal course of study such as that offered by the Transcultural Nursing Society[2] or some MSc courses in the UK as well as participation in local networks. The aim of such

[2] The Transcultural Nursing Society provides certificated courses and can be contacted via http://www.tcns.org

development is, at the very least, conscious competence in creating an approach to advanced assessment in which cultural values, beliefs, customs and practices are actively and thoughtfully considered in relation to the individual's health needs and problems and integrated into the practitioner's field of expertise.

Second, in working towards becoming culturally competent, advanced practitioners are able to act as agents for change. Initially this could be through acting as role models. McGee (2000), in a survey of nurses in acute hospital wards across four NHS trusts, found that staff lacked any kind of leadership or role models to help them provide culturally appropriate care. Of the 85 who participated, only 7 staff nurses had received any formal education about cultural dimensions of care and a further five had received some information during hospital induction courses. Consequently, the nurses' cultural knowledge and awareness were poor. Staff tended to conceptualise culture in either formulaic, stereotypical terms based on a narrow range of implications for staff such as which diet to order. Moreover, certain cultures, particularly those originating in South Asia, were pathologised because they were regarded either as obstacles that hindered patients' health or sources of difficulty for staff. In this context, the presence of an advanced practitioner who can work alongside staff to demonstrate culturally competent care, enable staff to develop their skills and constructively challenge negative attitudes, would provide a basis for improvement.

Third, advanced practitioners could develop local networks of professionals, service users and minority groups as a basis for providing staff development. David (1998), in her role as cultural liaison nurse, has shown how this networking can be harnessed to improve patient care. She developed a network spanning her health authority's catchment area that included health professionals, community services and agencies as diverse as the fire service and self-help groups. Through this network she was able to promote dialogue between groups that had previously never communicated with one another, for example bringing together members of a specific cultural group, health promotion officers, the fire service, safety officers and interpreters to educate people about fire and accident prevention. She was also able to draw on the network in providing training for staff in ways that provided both professional and lay perspectives. Her work demonstrates the potential in advanced practice roles for pioneering new ways of working that benefit both professionals and service users.

Culturally competent leadership and advanced practice

Cultural competence is a key element of leadership in advanced practice in two ways. First, advanced practitioners have a responsibility to facilitate culturally appropriate care within their field of practice as discussed above. Second, they have responsibilities within the organisation as a whole to encourage it to work towards cultural competence. This requires an understanding of the culture and subcultures of the organisation, how things are done and receptivity to change (McGee 1998). Hanson and Malone (2000: 293) argue that advanced practitioners should be able to assess the organisations within which they work to determine their 'level of commitment to diversity', sifting the rhetoric from the reality (Fig. 11.7). The place to begin this assessment is with the mission statement, goals, strategic plan and any other statements that the organisation makes about itself. Most organisations will wish to present themselves in a positive light, to give the appearance of being benign and non-discriminatory. However, comparisons between various organisational statements can reveal inconsistencies. A common discovery is that of short-term, selective engagements with culture (McGee 2000). For example, a trust may decide that there is a need to improve uptake of immunisation and vaccination among members of a minority ethnic group. A project is set up and a worker is appointed for a specified period of time to address this issue. Once the period of time has elapsed the project is closed. Such initiatives, whilst no doubt effective in achieving short-term goals, will not bring about change in the organisation. Even when staff attempt to bring about change, they may find their efforts thwarted by a lack of resources or the differing agendas of senior managers concerned with cost control and government-imposed targets. Thus it is instructive to examine the budget alongside organisational statements as a key indicator of the real priorities (Hanson & Malone 2000) (Fig. 11.7).

- What are the customs, rituals, traditions and symbols?
- Who is regarded as a hero/heroine and why?
- What are relationships like between staff and managers?
- What observations can be made about organisational values?

- What statements does the organisation make about itself and what are its true priorities?
- How does the organisation respond to racism?
- What communication systems are in place and are they effective?

Fig. 11.7   Assessing organisational commitment to diversity.

A second element in the assessment is the behaviour of staff. Most organisations will have policies and procedures dealing with what it regards as acceptable behaviour and what it will do when individuals transgress. One example is racism, harassment and prejudice. Numerous research reports have shown that these types of behaviour are taking place in healthcare settings even though such activities are illegal. The Department of Health (DoH 1998) introduced a strategy for tackling racial harassment and set out the action that was to be taken against those who behaved in this way. However, there is also evidence that social processes in the workplace allow racism to go unchecked. McGee (2000) found that recognising or reporting racist behaviour created dilemmas for nurses who feared reprisals from colleagues and lack of support from senior staff. Nurses did not know how to deal with racism and, therefore, resorted to punishing patients who, in their view, behaved badly or they simply turned a blind eye. Thus it is useful to ascertain if and how the organisation responds to racism or other discriminatory behaviour.

A third element to assess is the communications network. The organisation will have formal channels in place to cascade information and instructions to staff, but it should also have in place systems by which feedback is presented to senior managers. The effectiveness of these systems may vary but the advanced practitioner will need to become adept at using them to communicate with staff within and outside the organisation. Opportunities for training, such as courses in handling the media, will be important in communicating the relevance of cultural competence, educating staff, patients and the public on this issue.

Conclusion

This chapter has discussed a range of issues about cultural competence and advanced practice. In a culturally diverse society such as that of the UK the advanced practitioner must demonstrate the ability to meet the cultural needs of patients in relation to their health. Services that are appropriate and accessible are likely to be used more often and encourage users to seek help early. There is still a great deal of work to be done in making culturally competent care a reality but it is hoped that the following questions will help in nurses developing advanced practice in ways that reflect the diversity of local populations.

? **Key questions for Chapter 11**

In your field of practice:

(1) What strategies can be used to compile a database of the local client populations served by your field of practice?
(2) Which skills are needed to carry out this strategy and how might the advanced practitioner acquire these?
(3) How can the advanced practitioner promote the development of socially embedded expertise at both team level and in the organisation as a whole?

References

Ahmad,W. (ed.) (2000) *Ethnicity, Disability and Chronic Illness*. Buckingham: Open University Press.

Ahmad, W. & Atkin, K. (1996) (eds) *'Race' and Community Care*. Buckingham: Open University Press.

Andrews, M. & Boyle, J. (1999) *Transcultural Concepts in Nursing Care*, 3rd edn. Philadelphia: Lippincott.

Andrews, M. (2000) Transcultural considerations in assessment. In: *Physical Examination and Health Assessment* (ed. C. Jarvis), pp. 45–56, Philadelphia: W.B. Saunders.

Balarajan, R. & Raleigh, V. (1995) *Ethnicity and Health in England*. London: NHS Ethnic Health Unit/HMSO.

Beishon, S., Virdee, S. & Hagell, A. (1995) *Nursing in a Multi-Ethnic NHS*. London: Policy Studies Institute.

Benner, P., Tanner, C. & Chesla, C. (1996) *Expertise in Nursing Practice: Caring, Clinical Judgement and Ethics*. New York: Springer.

Brechin, A., Brown, H. & Eby, M. (eds) (2000) *Critical Practice in Health and Social Care*. London: Sage/Open University.

Campinha-Bacote, J. (1988) Culturalogical assessment: an important factor in psychiatric consultation liaison nursing. *Archives of Psychiatric Nursing*, 2(4): 244–50.

Campinha-Bacote, J. (1994a) *The Process of Competence in Health Care: A Culturally Competent Model of Care*, 2nd edn. Ohio: Transcultural CARE Associates.

Campinha-Bacote, J. (1994b) Cultural competence in psychiatric mental health nursing. *Nursing Clinics of North America*, 29 (1): 1–8.

Campinha-Bacote, J. (1995) The quest for cultural competence in nursing care. *Nursing Forum*, 30 (4): 19–25.

Campinha-Bacote, J. (1996) A culturally competent model of nursing management. *Surgical Services Management*, 2 (5): 22–5.

Cortis, J. (1998) The experience of nursing care by Pakistani (Urdu speaking) patients in later life in Dewsbury, West Yorkshire. Paper presented at 'What works': Research and Practice in Nursing, Midwifery and Health Visiting Conference, Leeds, June.

Darr, A. (1998) *Improving the Recruitment and Retention of Asian Students on Nursing, Midwifery, Radiography and Physiotherapy Courses: A Qualitative Research Study*. Report available from University of Bradford, School of Health Studies.

David, M. (1998) Cultural awareness and customer care. In: *Advanced and Specialist Nursing Practice* (eds G. Castledine & P. McGee), pp. 158–62. Oxford: Blackwell Science.

De Santis, L. (1994) Making anthropology clinically relevant to nursing care. *Journal of Advanced Nursing*, 20(4): 707–15.

DoH (1998) *Tackling Racial Harassment in the NHS: A Plan for Action*. Wetherby: DoH.

DoH (1999) *Making a Difference: Strengthening the Nursing, Midwifery and Health Visiting Contribution to Health and Healthcare*. London: DoH.

DoH (2001) *Modern Standards and Services Models. National Service Framework: Older People*. London: DoH.

Echols, J. (1998) Cultural assessment. In: *Health Assessment and Physical Examination* (ed. M.E.Z. Estes), pp. 101–27. Albany: Delmar.

Erens, B., Primatesta, P. & Prior, G. (2001) *Health Survey for England: The Health of Minority Ethnic Groups '99*. London: Joint Health Surveys Unit, National Centre for Social Research.

Estes, M.E.Z. (1998) (ed) *Health Assessment and Physical Examination*. Albany: Delmar.

Evers, H., Badger, F., Cameron, E. & Atkin, K. (1988) *Community Care Working Papers*. Birmingham: Department of Social Medicine, University of Birmingham.

Hanson, C. & Malone, B. (2000) Leadership: empowerment, change agency and activism. In *Advanced Nursing Practice: An Integrative Approach* (eds A. Hamric, J. Spross & C. Hanson), pp. 279–314. Philadelphia: W.B. Saunders.

Hofstede, G. (1994) *Culture and Organisations: Software of the Mind. Intercultural Co-operation and its Importance for Survival*. London: Harper Collins.

Home Office (1999) *The Stephen Lawrence Inquiry. Report of an Inquiry by Sir William Macpherson of Cluny*. London: The Stationery Office.

Kelleher, D. & Hillier, S. (eds)(1996) R*esearching Cultural Differences in Health*. London: Routledge.

Leininger, M. (1995) *Transcultural Nursing: Concepts, Theories and Practices*, 2nd edn. New York: McGraw-Hill.

Lilyman, S. (1998) Assessing competence. In: *Advanced and Specialist Nursing Practice* (eds G. Castledine & P. McGee), pp. 119–32. Oxford: Blackwell Science.

Lipson, J. & Steiger, N. (1996) *Self Care in a Multicultural Context*. Thousand Oaks, CA: Sage.

Malone, B. (1993) Caring for culturally diverse racial groups: an administrative matter. *Nursing Administration Quarterly*, 17 (2): 21–9.

McGee, P. (1998) *Models of Nursing in Practice: A Pattern for Practical Care*. Cheltenham: Stanley Thornes.

McGee, P. (1999) Meeting the needs of homeless people: the St John Ambulance mobile service. *Nursing Standard*, 13 (42): 38–40.

McGee, P. (2000) Culturally-sensitive nursing care: a critique. Unpublished PhD thesis, University of Central England.

Mendyka, B. (2000) Exploring culture in nursing: a theory-driven practice. *Holistic Nursing Practice*, 15 (1): 32–41.

NAHA (National Association of Health Authorities) (1988) *Action Not Words: A Strategy to Improve Health Services for Black and Minority Ethnic groups*. Birmingham: NAHA.

Nazroo, J. (1997) Health and health services. In: *Ethnic Minorities in Britain: Diversity and Disadvantage. The Fourth National Survey of Ethnic Minorities* (eds T. Modood & R. Berthoud), pp. 224–58. London: Policy Studies Institute.

Notter, J. & Klem, R. (2001) *Recruitment and Retention in Nursing and Professions Allied to Medicine of Individuals from Black and Minority Ethnic Communities*. Birmingham: Health and Social Care Research Centre, University of Central England.

Paniagua, F. (1994) *Assessing and Treating Culturally Diverse Clients: A Practical Guide*. Thousand Oaks, CA: Sage.

Papadopoulos, I. (2002) Promoting cultural competence with cancer patients. Conference paper published in *Culturally Competent Healthcare. Do we Understand It? How Do We Do It?* Proceedings of the Fourth National Conference of the Transcultural Nursing and Healthcare Association in partnership with the Research Centre for Transcultural Studies in Health, Middlesex University and the Foundation of Nursing Studies. Birmingham: Health and Social Care Research Centre, University of Central England.

Ramsden, I. (1995) Cultural Safety: Implementing the Concepts. Paper presented at the Social Force of Nursing and Midwifery Conference, James Cook Hotel, Wellington, New Zealand.

Rooda, L. (1992) The development of a conceptual model for multicultural nursing. *Journal of Holistic Nursing*, 10 (4): 337–47.

Roper, N., Logan, W. & Tierney, A. (1990) *The Elements of Nursing*, 3rd edn. Edinburgh: Churchill Livingstone.

Salimbene, S. (1999) Cultural competence: a priority for performance improvement action. *Journal of Nursing Care Quality*, 13 (3): 23–35.

Sands, R. & Hale, S. (1987) Enhancing cultural sensitivity in clinical practice. *Journal of the National Black Nurses' Association*, 2 (1): 54–63.

St Clair, A. & McKenry, L. (1999) Preparing culturally competent practitioners. *Journal of Nursing Education*, 38 (5): pp 228–34.

UKCC (1994) *The Future of Professional Practice – The Council's Standards for Education and Practice following Registration*. London: UKCC.

UKCC (1999) *A Higher Level of Practice. Report on the Consultation on the UKCC's Proposals for a Revised Regulatory Framework for Post-registration Clinical Practice*. London: UKCC.

Chapter 12

International Perspectives on Advanced Practice

Paula McGee

Introduction

Advanced nursing is a concept that began in the USA in response to a number of factors. These included addressing concerns about quality of care by developing new nursing roles such as that of clinical nurse specialist in which enhanced expertise and experience could be harnessed to improve practice. Changes in medical technology, for example the introduction of anaesthetics, provided other opportunities particularly in caring for the wounded in war zones. Nurses working in such environments acquired an expanded repertoire of clinical skills. On their return to civilian life, their evident expertise challenged the accepted scope of nursing practice. When a shortage of doctors in primary care meant that many, particularly rural, populations were underserved, nurses with enhanced expertise were able to develop new, community-based roles in an effort to address this situation (Menard 1987; Bigbee & Amidi-Nouri 2002).

Advanced practice must also be seen within the changing face and spiralling costs of American healthcare in which individuals are expected to have health insurance. A substantial number are unable to afford this and thus have limited access to healthcare or none at all. For these people there are two insurance schemes funded by the federal (national) government. Medicare covers about 40 million adults aged over 65 and some younger people with disabilities or end-stage renal disease provided they or their spouses have worked for at least ten years in jobs covered by the Medicare scheme. Medicaid provides insurance for about 34 million people on low incomes, but recent changes in funding arrangements have reduced the amount paid to each state and allowed state governments more freedom to decide who is eligible for support. There are now concerns that many children, pregnant women, elderly people in nursing homes and some disabled people may lose insurance cover and join the existing 42% of people in poverty who have no health insurance cover. In addition, reductions in federal funding have reduced the payments to doctors, making some of them reluctant to take on Medicaid patients, and the cumbersome bureaucracy (up to 30 pages in some states) associated with the scheme and designed to reduce fraud deters many others (Twentieth Century Fund 2002). In this context, advanced practice is as much about changing social and political agendas as it is about professional expertise. Advanced practice has become a way of increasing access to healthcare for the poor and for those who live in remote areas.

From this background, nurses in the USA have continued work on the concept of advanced practice, developing and diversifying their roles. Their ideas have attracted considerable interest from many different countries and societies faced with similar problems in meeting the healthcare needs of their populations. This chapter examines some of the key issues in this global focus on advanced practice. The chapter begins by examining the perspective of the World Health Organisation (WHO) that has an international responsibility for setting agendas for healthcare and nursing. This is followed by a discussion that draws on reports from the USA, Canada, Australia, Ireland, the Philippines, Fiji and South Africa: countries that have all either developed or are in the process of developing their own approaches to advanced practice. This discussion reveals a number of issues of shared concern. First, there are issues about developing an internationally agreed definition and scope of advanced practice that also meets the requirements of nursing in individual countries. Second, there are issues in determining the competence of advanced practitioners that are closely allied to the third factor, clarifying work and role activities. Fourth, factors concerning the level of preparation and education required for advanced practice are discussed. Finally, the interface between advanced nursing practice and that of medicine are addressed. The chapter draws to a close with an outline of the work of the international advanced practice network.

A global agenda for nursing

The report of the Global Advisory Group on Nursing and Midwifery (WHO 2000) stated that nursing services are 'a critical component of the infrastructure for providing essential health services' because 'nursing and midwifery personnel constitute the largest component of the health workforce and deliver, or supervise, most of the health services provided worldwide'. This means that nursing, through sheer force of numbers, is regarded as having the potential for a high profile in targeting many of the current global concerns about the provision of healthcare. These concerns focus on improving access to quality primary healthcare by developing new ways of community-based working that serve to meet the increased need for home care and which can form part of the public health strategies required to combat escalating communicable diseases especially tuberculosis, malaria and HIV/AIDS (Schober 2002).

The Advisory Group went on to recommend that

- WHO should provide support in strengthening the capacity of ministries of health to review national health policies, plans and systems, and to enhance the contribution of the nursing and midwifery services in meeting the needs of vulnerable and marginalized populations.
- considering the critical shortage of nurses and midwives globally, WHO should review national efforts for health workforce planning and identify models appropriate to different health systems in order to ensure that human resources are more relevant to the actual needs of the service and the population. This would include mechanisms for the dissemination of these models and the development of guidelines on the use of such models. (WHO 2000)

Advanced practice can be seen as one model whereby everyday healthcare needs of people can be met through the use of nursing expertise. Only patients who require more than that expertise are referred to a doctor (Smith 1995). Advanced practice is part of the frontline provision of health services that make creative use of nursing knowledge and skill. Advanced practice also provides opportunities for health systems to make the best use of doctors, allowing them to focus their attention on those who most need their help.

Definitions and scope of advanced practice

Approximately 30 countries are currently exploring or developing ideas about advanced practice in line with the recommendations made by WHO. These countries include several African states, Australia, those in the Caribbean, western Europe and those on the Pacific Rim such as Fiji, Taiwan, South Korea and Hong Kong. One of the challenges facing all these countries is that of defining advanced practice in a way that is meaningful and appropriate both within and between states. This has required considerable professional debate as the following examples show.

First, the American Nurses' Association (ANA) defined advanced practice as having three components: specialisation, expansion and advancement.

> Specialisation in concentrating or delimiting one's focus to part of the whole field of nursing. Expansion refers to the acquisition of new practice knowledge and skills, including the knowledge and skill that legitimise role autonomy within areas of practice that overlap traditional boundaries of medical practice. Advancement involves both specialisation and expansion and is characterised by the integration of a broad range of theoretical, research-based, and practical knowledge that occurs as part of graduate education in nursing. (ANA 1995: 14).

The term 'advanced nurse practitioner' is an umbrella term for nurses engaged primarily in clinical practice who have undergone master's level training to become clinical registered nurse anaesthetists, certified nurse midwives, clinical nurse specialists and nurse practitioners (Hamric 2000). These four roles have been designated as advanced by the ANA and by an increasing number of state practice Acts (Hamric 1998; Pearson 1999, 2000).

Second, in Ireland,

> advanced nursing and midwifery practice is carried out by autonomous practitioners who are competent, accountable and responsible for their own practice. They are highly experienced in clinical practice and educated to master's degree or higher. (National Council for the Professional Development of Nursing and Midwifery 2001)

Advanced practice is directed towards the promotion of wellness in diverse settings through the use of sophisticated nursing or midwifery skills. Expert and autonomous practice is at the centre of advanced nursing and midwifery but emphasis is also placed on the ability to envision new horizons in nursing or midwifery and work towards incorporating these into the care given to patients.

Finally, in Canada, advanced nursing practice is defined as that which improves access to integrated and effective healthcare. As in the USA, the title of advanced nurse practitioner is an umbrella term that

> describes an advanced level of nursing practice that maximises the use of in depth nursing knowledge and skill in meeting the healthcare needs of clients (individuals, families, groups, populations or entire communities). In this way advanced nursing practice extends the boundaries of nursing's scope of practice and contributes to nursing knowledge as well as the development and advancement of the profession. (Canadian Nurses Association 1999)

Advanced practice is based on initial nurse education but requires further preparation at postgraduate level and a wide range of experience (Locking-Cusolito 2000).

Comparison of these definitions shows an emergent agreement, between nurses in different countries and healthcare systems, that there is a form or level of practice that is beyond that of initial preparation and which is based on the integration of a wide range of theoretical and practical knowledge. All three definitions emphasise that this advanced level of practice is rooted in nursing, client-focused and directed towards health. These emphases are significant in distinguishing advanced nursing practice from the practice of medicine. Advanced practice is not a route to becoming a doctor. It is a new way of conceptualising practice that recognises the depth and potential of nursing and which directs the application of professional knowledge and skills towards the needs of the modern world. It reflects a 'way of thinking and viewing the world based on clinical knowledge rather than a composition of roles' (Davies & Hughes 1995). Such roles require certain qualities such as creativity and a pioneering spirit as well as demonstrative academic ability at master's degree level or above. Thus, being an advanced practitioner is about the type of person the nurse is as much as the professional knowledge and expertise an individual may possess. This agreed focus on clinical practice, master's level education, and developing new arenas for nursing as essential ingredients of advanced practice are reflected in the definition published by the International Council of Nurses (ICN). The Council states that a

> Nurse Practitioner/Advanced Practice Nurse is a registered nurse who has acquired the expert knowledge base, complex decision-making skills and clinical competencies for expanded practice, the characteristics of which are shaped by the context and/or country in which s/he is credentialed to practise. A master's degree is recommended for entry level. (ICN 2002)

The Council makes clear that this definition has to be examined in relation to local need but argues that it provides a basis for a unified way forward.

The Council elaborates on this definition by identifying factors that shape the scope of advanced practice in any country irrespective of the setting. In the Council's view the advanced practitioner should be an initial point of contact for clients wishing to access healthcare. Advanced practitioners should be able to assess the needs of those clients, and plan, implement and evaluate their care using a repertoire of knowledge and skills drawn from diverse sources and which exceeds that normally required for professional practice. Moreover, advanced practitioners should be able to practise autonomously and provide a source of expertise for other professionals who consult them for advice (Table 12.1).

Table 12.1   ICN criteria for advanced practice

The advanced practitioner:
• Integrates research, education, practice and management
• Has a high degree of professional autonomy and independent practice
• Involves case management/own caseload
• Requires advanced health assessment skills, decision-making skills and diagnostic reasoning skills
• Recognises advanced clinical competences
• Provides consultant services to health providers
• Includes the planning, implementation and evaluation of programmes
• Is recognised as first point of contact for clients

In addition to the general factors set out in Table 12.1, there should be country-specific regulatory mechanisms in place that provide advanced practitioners with the legal and professional rights to their professional titles and authority to function as autonomous professionals. Such authority should include the right to diagnose and treat illness and refer patients to other sources of help without the intervention of a third party such as a doctor (Table 12.2).

Table 12.2   ICN country-specific criteria for establishing advanced practice

There should be legislation and regulations in place that provide advanced practitioners with protected titles and the authority to:
• Diagnose
• Prescribe medication
• Prescribe treatment
• Refer clients to other professionals
• Admit patients to hospital

The definition and criteria for advanced practice provided by the Council represent partial progress. In returning to the three definitions examined earlier in this chapter it is evident even there that a number of issues remain unresolved. First, there are local inconsistencies in definition and scope of practice. Canada and the USA regard the term 'advanced practice' as an umbrella term that covers designated roles that include midwifery. In contrast, the Irish view is much broader and reflects a healthcare system in which midwifery is a separate profession. This raises concerns about the extent to which definitions and criteria for advanced nursing can be applied across professional boundaries or whether midwifery is in some way a special category.

Second, the emphasis on patient-centred and autonomous practice, in which the nurse is the first and possibly only point of contact with health services, may accurately reflect the ability of nurses to function in this way. However, it does not automatically follow that patients, families or communities regard this ability as meaningful or desirable. For advanced practice to be successful patients need to understand and feel confident that nurses can meet their needs. Advanced practice is, therefore, dependent on public education and acceptance. A similar point can be made about other professional groups, particularly medicine, that have traditionally held responsibility for the diagnosis and treatment of ill health and acted as gate-keepers to other sources of help. The development of new advanced roles must involve constructive dialogue in which the welfare and wishes of the patients remain a primary concern and in which revised lines of responsibility and accountability are clarified. Moreover, advanced practitioners must demonstrate that they have received the necessary preparation for new responsibilities and are competent in their performance (Turnberg *et al.* 1996).

Third, as the ICN has made clear, advanced practice requires the support of country-specific legislation that legitimises new ways of working. Such legislation should also require those who manage health services to put in place quality assurance systems in which standards for advanced practice are set and monitored alongside patient satisfaction (Schober 2002).

Work activities and competence

According to the American Nurses' Association (ANA 1996), the work activities of advanced nurses are 'a high level of expertise in the assessment, diagnosis and treatment of the complex responses of individuals, families or communities to actual or potential health problems, prevention of illness or injury, maintenance of wellness and provision of comfort.' Pearson (2000) supports this stance, adding that advanced practitioners optimise health and work to prevent illness and disability. In her view, this focus on health provides the basis for distinguishing advanced nurses from other professionals (Table 12.3).

The reality of working as an advanced practitioner reveals a rather different picture. An international survey of 81 advanced nurses from 39 countries showed that just over half were able to practice autonomously, only one-third had the right to diagnose or initiate treatment, and far fewer had any prescribing authority (Table 12.4).

Table 12.3   Characteristics of advanced practitioners

Advanced practitioners	Differences between advanced practitioners and other professionals
Diagnose and treat illness Initiate and advance medical treatment Advise on case management Prevent illness/disability and reduce recurrence Optimise health	Empower patients and families Coordinate use of community resources Promote wellness-oriented self-care Provide comprehensive health education Teach preventative health promotion activities Coordinate care Negotiate the healthcare system as patient advocates

Table 12.4   Survey of work roles (Nurse Practitioner/Advanced Practice Network 2001)

- 67% provided consultant services
- 60% provided research functions
- 59% acted as the first point of contact
- 51% had autonomy and independence
- 49% were responsible for planning, implementing and evaluation programmes
- 33% had the right to diagnose
- 30% had authority to prescribe treatment
- 30% were able to set up a private practice
- 23% had the authority to prescribe medicine

Moreover, even within a single country there can be considerable variation in practice because of difference in legislation, scope of practice and local circumstances (Tables 12.5, 12.6). To illustrate this point, in the USA each state has its own Nurse Practice Act and regulations concerning advanced practice. There are approximately 149,716 advanced practitioners, but numbers vary considerably across the country, with California having the highest number at 15,279 and Wyoming the least at 250 (all these figures show an increase over the previous year) (Pearson 2001, 2002). Variations

Table 12.5   Legislative control of advanced practice in the USA as at 2002 (Pearson 2001, 2002)

- In 25 (2001: 24) states, the title of Advanced Nurse Practitioner (which may include CNS, CNMs, CNAs etc.) is protected and the Board of Nursing is the sole authority in the scope of practice. There is no requirement for collaboration with/supervision by a physician
- In 13 (2001: 13) states, the Board of Nursing is the sole authority in the scope of practice but there is the requirement of collaboration with a physician
- In 6 (2001: 7) states the Board of Nursing is the sole authority in the scope of practice but there is the requirement of supervision by a physician
- In 6 (2001: 6) states the Board of Nursing and the Board of Medicine regulate the scope of practice
- In 1 state there is no separate legislation concerning advanced practice

Table 12.6   Prescriptive authority for advanced practice in the USA as at 2002 (Pearson, 2001, 2002)

- In 13 (2001: 12) states, advanced nurses can prescribe, including controlled substances, independently of a physician
- In 32 (2001: 31) states, advanced nurses can prescribe, including controlled substances, with some degree of supervision by a doctor
- In 6 (2001: 8) states, advanced nurses can prescribe, excluding controlled substances, with some degree of supervision by a doctor
- From 1999, advanced nurses were granted some form of prescribing authority in every state

in legislative control between states have considerable effect on the nature of advanced practice. For example, in Alaska an advanced nurse is defined as a registered nurse who because of specialised education and experience, is certified to perform acts of medical diagnosis and prescription and dispensing of medical, therapeutic or corrective measures under regulations adopted by the Board of Nursing which has sole regulatory responsibility. The Board recognises nurse practitioners and clinical nurse midwives as advanced nurses and there are separate rules governing certified registered nurse anaesthetists. Advanced practitioners must have a plan for consultation with, and referral of their patients to, a doctor. Certified nurse midwives can admit patients to the Alaska Native Hospital but others require a doctor to act as preceptor although there is no law that states this is necessary. Advanced practitioners can send bills for their services directly to insurers and are paid 80% of a doctor's fee. They also have independent prescribing authority, including controlled substances (Pearson 2002).

In contrast, in the state of Virginia, the Board of Nursing and the Board of Medicine govern regulation jointly. Nurse practitioners, certified nurse midwives, clinical nurse specialists and certified registered nurse anaesthetists are recognised as advanced practitioners. They must be certified and practise under medical direction and supervision. They must develop a practice agreement with the supervisor that must be approved by both boards. Advanced practitioners can send bills directly to insurers but are not always paid, as they are not mandated care providers. When they are paid, certified nurse midwives, family nurse practitioners and psychiatric nurse practitioners are paid the same as doctors. They may prescribe, including controlled drugs, using written protocols agreed with the supervisor as part of the practice agreement submitted by that person to the joint boards, and the name and address of the supervising physician must be given with the prescription (Pearson 2002).

Thus in Alaska the Board of Nursing has sole control of and responsibility for advanced nursing. The Board determines who is competent to practise and makes clear that advanced nurses can function autonomously, diagnose, treat illnesses and in some circumstances admit patients to hospital. In Virginia, advanced nurses are not so independent and are subject to both medical supervision and the supervision of the Board of Nursing.

Developments in Ireland provide yet another approach that places responsibilities on managers. The National Council for the Professional Development of Nursing and

Midwifery (2001) states that the establishment of any advanced nursing or midwifery post is dependent on two factors. First, the managers responsible must present a case for the post highlighting the healthcare need and defining the role. They must also put in place systems that will ensure good practice, accept responsibility for vicarious liability and identify and resource implications. Second, the individual practitioner must apply to the Council for accreditation, presenting, with the managers, a detailed portfolio of the area of practice, documentary description of the skills involved and evidence of both research activities and participation in professional activities. Whilst these examples may well arise because of local circumstances, each provides a potential model for future exploration and research.

Interface with medicine

Nursing theorists are keen to point out that advanced practice is about developing nursing and not about taking over medical work. However, the literature indicates an uneasy relationship between the two disciplines. A case study from South Africa presents an account of an advanced nurse working in primary care who consulted a doctor after discovering that a patient had a heart murmur. The doctor responded in a hostile manner, challenging the nurse's right to make such a diagnosis. The study demonstrated not only the way in which hostility can flare up in everyday situations but also how isolated, and therefore vulnerable, that particular nurse was. Without an effective support system and clearly designated lines of responsibility she found herself dealing with the situation alone (May 1995).

Similar difficulties have been reported in the USA, where, as the advanced role has moved from rural into urban and acute hospital environments, doctors began to feel quite threatened. It must be emphasised that not everyone shared this sense of threat. Some were very supportive, but as a body, doctors responded rather negatively to advanced practice. Pearson (2001) reports that doctors have seen their professional power challenged through the introduction of managed care, the development of Internet-based systems that allow patients to evaluate practitioners online and increasing patient power. In this context, advanced practice can be regarded as yet another source of threat to which the American Medical Association (AMA) has responded with 'an intensive on-line advocacy campaign to help medical societies defeat state and national legislation that increases the professional autonomy of APNs [advanced practice nurses] and other providers. The AMA's goal is to kill legislation that does not allow ultimate physician control' (Pearson 2001).

Given this potential for serious interprofessional conflict it is useful to examine an alternative approach to the introduction of advanced practice. Like the USA, Australia has also experienced difficulties in recruiting doctors to work in remote and rural areas. Nurses working in these settings provide the only access to healthcare and each state has its own regulations about the nature of nursing practice. Moreover, their very isolation and the nature of the communities they serve (and often belong to through family or marriage), requires that remote and rural nurses practise outside normal professional boundaries (Siegloff 1995; Keyzer 1997). Nurses in Australia have, therefore, examined the usefulness of advanced practice in their healthcare system.

For example, in 1992 the New South Wales (NSW) Department of Health invited the NSW Nurses' Association to submit a discussion paper on advanced roles. This paper put forward the notion that advanced practice is carried out by 'a registered nurse who practises in an expanded role with professional autonomy in a work setting in which the nurse has the freedom to make discretionary and binding decisions consistent with the nurse's scope of practice and the freedom to act on those decisions' (Appel & Malcolm 1999). This definition provoked a hostile response from doctors and led to the setting up of a multidisciplinary working party that included medical practitioners who established pilot projects in remote, rural and urban settings. The outcome of these projects was a list of 15 recommendations based on the recognition that advanced practitioners were legitimate healthcare providers and which included limited prescribing rights, referral rights (except to specialist doctors) and changes in legislation to allow the role to develop according to local needs (Appel & Malcolm 1999).

This example demonstrates that confrontation with medical practitioners is not inevitable and can be offset by involving medical practitioners in the development of advanced nursing practice, listening to their concerns and valuing their professional points of view. It is justifiable and appropriate that they should ask searching questions about the capacity of advanced practice to provide accurate assessment of and treatment for common illnesses. Medical practitioners recognise that the complexity of modern healthcare and their shortage of numbers, when compared with nursing, require them to address how best to make use of their skills (BMA 2002). The Australian example shows that advanced practice can coexist with medicine and need not be perceived as a threat.

Preparation and level of education among nurses

The ICN (2002) statement on advanced practice makes clear that some form of preparation beyond initial qualification is essential and recommends that this should be at master's level or above. The American Nurses' Association, the Canadian Nurses' Association, National Council for the Professional Development of Nursing and Midwifery in Ireland and nursing organisations in other countries as well as theorists such as Hamric (2000) support this recommendation as one of the primary criteria for advanced practice. The international survey undertaken by the Nurse Practitioner/Advanced Practice Network (2001) found that 82% (n = 81) of respondents reported having a nursing role that required education beyond initial qualification. A total of 69% reported that they had formal educational programmes preparing advanced nurses in their country; and 64% reported that this education led to a recognised degree. Finally, 79% reported that their country had programmes that were accredited or approved.

The survey report gave no indication of the academic status of initial nurse education in the respondents' countries. Where entry to the profession is already at first-degree level, as for example in the USA, a master's degree can be regarded as a reasonable way of demonstrating both academic and professional development. However, this situation is not universal. For example, the school of nursing at Nacuva, Fiji, launched its first nursing degree in 2002. In the first cohort of 25 students were 11 members of the school staff. According to the Fijian government, upgrading the education of staff was an essential precursor to the development of any courses leading to advanced or specialist qualifications (Fiji Government On Line 2002). In a paper from the Philippines, Stark *et al.* (1999) question the appropriateness of the master's degree, particularly in developing countries in which the only healthcare available to the majority of the population is that provided by nurses. They argue that some poorer countries may not be able to afford postgraduate education for these nurses. Even where such courses are possible, there will be those who lack the formal entry requirements. What, they ask, should happen to those who lack formal qualifications but who are fulfilling a much-needed role?

To be fair, Stark *et al.*'s (1999) concerns are pertinent to all countries embarking on or considering the introduction of advanced practice. In each case there is likely to be a workforce of experienced nurses performing essential and effective services. Some of these nurses may well be utilising advanced skills and acting as the first or only point of contact with healthcare. There are undoubtedly professional, ethical and financial issues to be addressed in this situation in ways that value that contribution of such nurses and enable them to continue to meet the needs of patients.

Conclusion

This chapter has examined advanced practice from a global perspective. There are currently about 30 countries that have either introduced or are exploring this approach to nursing. In doing so, those responsible for healthcare must develop affordable approaches that meet local needs and in which standards and work roles are agreed. Such approaches must also take account of developments at international level. The Advanced Practice Network was launched at the 8th International Conference of Nurse Practitioners in San Diego, California, in 2000, under the auspices of the ICN with a view to facilitating dialogue and collaboration at international level. The forum can be accessed via the Internet at http://www.icn.ch/networks or via the following address:

Advanced Practice Network
International Council of Nurses
3 Place Jean-Marteau
1201 – Geneva
Switzerland

? Key questions for Chapter 12

In your field of practice:

(1) How can the public be prepared for and informed about the introduction of advanced practitioners as the first point of contact with the health services?
(2) What approaches could be used in your workplace to gain support from medical colleagues for the introduction of advanced practice roles?
(3) What other roles, besides that of advanced practice, could be developed to promote inclusive approaches to the provision of healthcare?

References

ANA (1995) *Nursings Social Policy Statement.* Washington, DC: ANA.
ANA (1996) *Scope and Standards of Advanced Practice Registered Nursing.* Washington, DC: ANA.
Appel, A.L. & Malcolm, P. (1999) The struggle for recognition: the nurse practitioner in New South Wales, Australia. *Clinical Nurse Specialist*, 13 (5): 236–41.
Bigbee, J. & Amidi-Nouri, A. (2002) History and evolution of advanced nursing practice. In: *Advanced Nursing Practice: An Integrative Approach*, 2nd edn (eds A. Hamric, J. Spross & C. Hanson), pp. 3–32. Philadelphia: W.B. Saunders.
BMA (2002) The future healthcare workforce. HPERU Discussion Paper 9. Available at http://www.bma.org.uk (accessed March 2002).
Canadian Nurses' Association (1999) http://can-nurses.ca (accessed September).
Davies, B. & Hughes, A. (1995) Clarification of advanced nursing practice: characteristics and competencies. *Clinical Nurse Specialist*, 9 (3): 156–60,166.
Fiji Government On Line (2002) http://www.fiji.gov.fj (accessed September 2002).
Hamric, A. (1998) Historical and current developments in specialist and advanced practice in North America. In: *Advanced and Specialist Nursing Practice* (eds G. Castledine & P. McGee), pp. 55–70. Oxford: Blackwell Science.
Hamric, A. (2000) A definition of advanced nursing practice. In: *Advanced Nursing Practice: An Integrative Approach*, 2nd edn (eds A. Hamric, J. Spross & C. Hanson), pp. 53–73. Philadelphia: W.B. Saunders.
ICN (2002) http://icn.org (accessed September 2002).
Keyzer, D. (1997) Working together: the advanced rural nurse practitioner and the rural doctor. *Australian Journal of Rural Health*, 5 (4): 184–9.
Locking-Cusolito, H. (2000) Advanced practice nurses and their role in nephrology settings. *Nephrology Nursing Journal*, 27 (2): 245–7.
May, W.V. (1995) A case study of primary health care practice in a selected urban area in South Africa. *Curationis*, 18 (2): 28–32.
Menard, S. (1987) The CNS: historical perspectives. In: *The Clinical Nurse Specialist: Perspectives on Practice* (ed. S. Menard), pp. 1–8. New York: John Wiley.
National Council for the Professional Development of Nursing and Midwifery (2001) *Framework for the Establishment of Advanced Nurse and Advanced Practitioner Posts.* Dublin: An Bord Altranais. Available at www.nursingboard.ie (accessed September 2002).
Nurse Practitioner/Advanced Practice Network (2001) www.icn.ch/networks (accessed September 2002).

Pearson, L. (1999) Annual update. How each state stands on legislative issues affecting advanced nursing practice. *The Nurse Practitioner: The American Journal of Primary Health Care*, 24 (1): 16–19, 23–4, 27–8, 30, 35–8, 40, 42, 45–6, 49–50, 52, 55, 60, 62, 67–70, 73–4, 79–80, 83.

Pearson, L. (2000) Annual legislative update. How each state stands on legislative issues affecting advanced nursing practice. *The Nurse Practitioner: The American Journal of Primary Health Care*, 25 (1): 16–18, 21, 25–6, 27–8, 31–33, 36–8, 41–2, 44–8, 51–2, 54–6, 63, 67–8.

Pearson, L. (2001) Annual legislative update. How each state stands on legislative issues affecting advanced nursing practice. *The Nurse Practitioner*, 26 (1): 7, 11–15, 17–18, 21–27, 28, 31–8, 47–54, 57.

Pearson, L. (2002) Fourteenth annual legislative update. How each state stands on legislative issues affecting advanced nursing practice. *The Nurse Practitioner*, 27 (1): 10–12, 15, 19–20, 22–4, 26–30, 33–4, 37–40, 43, 52.

Schober, M. (2002) Global development of nurse practitioner/advanced practice roles. Paper presented at the RCN Valuing Diversity: Nurse Practitioners in the 21st Century Conference, Manchester, September.

Siegloff, L.H. (1995) The nurse practitioner project, Wilcannia: moving from anecdotes to evidence. *Australian Journal of Rural Health*, 3 (3): 114–21.

Smith, M. (1995) The core of advanced nursing practice. *Nursing Science Quarterly*, 8 (1): 2–3.

Stark, R., Nair, N.V.K. & Omi, S. (1999) Nurse practitioners in developing countries: some ethical considerations. *Nursing Ethics*, 6 (4): 273–7.

Turnberg, L., Evans, J., Cameron, I., Ward, J., London, J., Hancock, C. & Winder, E. (1996) Skillsharing. Joint statement from the Royal College of Physicians of London and the Royal College of Nursing. *Journal of the Royal College of Physicians of London*, 30 (1): 57.

Twentieth Century Fund (2002) Available at http://www.tcf.org/ (accessed September 2002).

WHO (2000) *Global Advisory Group on Nursing and Midwifery. Report of the 6th Meeting*. Geneva: WHO. Available at www.who.org (accessed September 2002).

Chapter 13

Advanced Nursing Practice and the Interface with Medicine in the UK

Alison Gidlow and Brian Ellis

Introduction

The view of advanced practice put forward in this book is rooted firmly in nursing and the delivery of direct care to patients by professionally mature practitioners whose extensive knowledge and skill enable them to develop new directions. Inevitably elements of their knowledge and skill will require them to undertake activities that may also be performed by other health professionals including doctors. In other instances the advanced nature of their role can serve to highlight the common ground that exists between senior professionals (Hunsberger *et al.* 1992). In neither case does this mean that advanced practitioners are encroaching on the domains of others. Health professionals, in particular those in nursing and medicine, need to be clear that advanced nursing practice is not an alternative route into the practice of medicine. This is an important statement because, as has been argued in Chapter 12 of this book, there is potential for serious interprofessional conflict that can be averted through constructive collaboration in which the concerns and views of nurses and doctors are openly shared and valued.

This chapter examines the interface between advanced nursing and medicine from the perspectives of an advanced practitioner and a medical consultant. It begins with a discussion of the nurse–doctor partnership and the opportunities afforded by advanced practice for this to enter a new phase based on equality. This is followed by a discussion of the differences in focus between the holistic approach used in advanced nursing, practice and the more complaint-oriented direction of medicine. It is argued that the holistic approach has contributed to more seamless care than can be achieved by junior medical staff who are required to change their posting every few months. Collaboration between advanced nursing and medicine is the cornerstone for success. Collaboration requires mutual respect and a valuing of the other's expertise that fosters constructive working relationships and pre-empts confrontation. The basis for such collaboration in one work setting is presented in this chapter as an illustration of the ways in which good practice can be developed.

The interface between nursing and medicine

The NHS reforms of recent years (DoH 1997a, 1999a, 2000a) have not only given rise to the development of advanced nursing roles, but have also disrupted the historic pattern of doctor–nurse interaction. The doctor–nurse divide is now being challenged, as never before, following recognition that realignment of the medical and nursing professions is an essential component of the future NHS. Nurses working at an advanced level now practise within a variety of settings: acute care; A&E outpatient clinics; GP practices; walk-in centres and NHS Direct. These nurses have changed the traditional boundaries between nursing and medicine. The key to a successful working partnership between nursing and medicine is collaboration, not confrontation. Not only is there increasing overlap between the professions in terms of care provision, but there are also clear distinctions between advanced nursing practice and medicine. These distinctions, and the benefits to patient care that the nursing skills within such roles bring, need to be clearly articulated and demonstrated in order to silence those critics who maintain that such roles are simply doctor substitution or 'nurses practising medicine' (Pearson 1996; Alcolado 2000).

Nurses practising at an advanced level combine nursing and medical roles, thus bringing medicine into nursing, and bringing nursing and medicine together. Rather than a doctor substitute, this combination of roles has constituted a new 'hybrid' health worker (Reveley & Haigh 2001). The traditionally dominant position of medicine is slowly giving way, as the combination of patient needs, manpower and resource factors bring about reform. The increased interchangeability between the professions also signals a reduced reliance on medicine. In addition to this change in culture within the NHS, there has been a much greater emphasis on multi-professional teamworking (English 1997). This is strongly supported by a government that urges greater interprofessional collaboration (DoH 2000a,b). According to the Royal College of Physicians (2000): 'Increasingly healthcare is delivered by a multi-professional team, and the consultant is not always the leader of the team … there has been a change in the mindset of most doctors, who now accept that the mode of delivery of healthcare has to change if it is to improve, as it must.'

There is now the potential for a new nurse–doctor partnership to emerge on an equal footing. This will evolve ideally into a patient–nurse–doctor triad. That this potential exists is the result of a dramatic shift in the doctor–nurse relationship during the past 30 years. Stein *et al.* (1990) identified a number of social changes that had led to alterations in the relationship. These included: a decline in public esteem for doctors, with medical infallibility increasingly challenged in the hospital and courtroom; stereotypical roles of male dominance and female passivity not surviving owing to the burgeoning numbers of women entering the medical profession; and a gradual fading of the role of the nurse as handmaiden with increasing numbers of nurses taking greater responsibility in healthcare provision. As a result of these changes, there has emerged the opportunity for greater nursing autonomy and collaborative practice options. As nurses become more involved in nurse-led interventions, such as assessment clinics and chronic disease management, referring aspects of clinical care that can be managed well by appropriately educated nurses to medical colleagues is uneconomical and inefficient. The approach of the UKCC in the Scope of Professional Practice (UKCC 1992) document was about moving away from a list of nursing and medical tasks. The emphasis was on assessing the needs of the patient and ensuring that whoever carried out the procedure was competent to do so.

Reveley *et al.* (2001) make the distinction between extending and expanding nursing roles. Nurses extending their roles are taking on tasks delegated by doctors and require close supervision from doctors. This reduces autonomy and leaves nurses in a position of responsibility without authority. These nurses are susceptible to the vagaries of a more powerful profession and a hierarchical relationship is maintained. However, nurses expanding their role are entering into a partnership with patients and doctors, having responsibility for a caseload, admitting and discharging patients from healthcare systems, referring to other agencies, and have involvement in teaching junior doctors about healthcare. This role allows the nurse–patient partnership to become the alternative to the doctor–patient partnership. The nursing profession needs to make it clear that it is the latter role that is espoused for advanced nursing practice.

Walsh (2001) suggests that medical staff will tend to interpret the advanced nursing concept differently from nurses and therefore both parties have to clarify and understand each other's perceptions of the concept if agreement is to be reached. Medicine has to relinquish a degree of power if advanced nursing practice is to develop. Healthcare provided by doctors is used as the gold standard for healthcare delivery and, as Reveley (1999a) avers, some take it for granted that 'damage to patients' will occur if nurses are used as substitutes for doctors. For this reason it is important that care provision is not delegated from doctors to nurses in an ad hoc fashion. It is imperative that nurses expanding their role into the domain of medicine, for example history-taking, physical examination, differential diagnosis and clinical decision-making, have gained the necessary knowledge and skills to perform these functions competently. The goal has to be shared responsibility for patient care, with both doctors and nurses administering therapy, monitoring and managing treatment and disease effects and, in addition, providing psychological support. Knowledge and insights need to be shared, contributing to the overall plan of care and leading to a productive nurse–doctor relationship. In the early 1990s, Henry (1994) urged nursing and medicine to recognise that the complexities of healthcare decisions and the technologies involved require the insight of both doctors and nurses working interdependently. This still holds true for healthcare provision today.

Distinctions between advanced nursing practice and medicine

Some attempts to understand the growth of advanced nursing practice on the boundaries of nursing and medicine have endeavoured to reduce both to a simple list of tasks, and then decide who does what. For instance, Richardson and Maynard (1995) stated that studies suggested that between 30% and 70% of doctors' tasks could be carried out by nurses, but warned that many of these studies lacked external validity. However, Barton *et al.* (1999) asserted that the labelling of tasks as nursing or medical was historically dated. Although it is true to say that nurses practising at an advanced level undertake care previously only located within the domain of medicine, it is the nursing focus brought to the consultation that patients value (NHS Executive, 1996; Centre for Health Services Research 1998; Reveley 1998).

The distinctions between the medical and nursing approaches are apparent in patient perceptions. Reveley (1999b), Kinnersley *et al.* (2000) and Horrocks *et al.* (2002) found that the difference in consultations between nurses and GPs centred around time and the perception of not feeling rushed, and interpersonal skills such as listening, talking, giving full explanations and being easy to talk to. In addition, the patients showed that they valued the clinical competence demonstrated by the nurse. Research by Williams (1998) found nurse qualities appreciated by patients to be: being careful, gentle, kind, friendly, respectful, attentive and considerate. Such qualities are similar to the 'comfort work' described by Strauss *et al.* (1985). Patients can be fearful of the implications of a diagnosis and the possibility of pain during treatment. According to Strauss *et al.* (1985), 'failure to do comfort work to patients' satisfaction is a major source of their anger and frustration and leads to complaints and accusations of incompetence or negligence'.

Nurses practising at an advanced level make diagnosis and treatment decisions, consult with medical colleagues and refer to other healthcare or social agencies as appropriate. Some of these skills are traditionally perceived as being within the domain of medicine, and it could be argued that these nurses are practising in a way more affiliated to medicine than nursing. However, Walsh (2001) suggests that the distinction between the ways in which the two professions practise can be seen by considering the direct approach of medicine, which focuses on the chief complaint and works through to a diagnosis via history-taking and physical examination. By comparison, the nursing approach is much more concerned with the human response to health and illness and makes a more holistic assessment which incorporates biological, sociological, psychological, cultural and family factors. Inui (1994) believes that the medical profession has tended to look at its role too narrowly by simply sifting through symptoms, making a diagnosis, prescribing a treatment and determining medical progress. He suggests that 'social healing' or 'tender loving care' is often tacked on only as an adjunct, if at all.

Advanced nursing roles are well-received by patients because they combine the skills traditionally associated with nursing with those associated with medicine, such as physical assessment and diagnosis. Evaluation has found consultations with nurses provide comparable outcomes to those with doctors, and high levels of patient satisfaction (Kinnersley *et al.* 2000; Shum *et al.* 2000). Horrocks *et al.* (2002), in a systematic review of the literature, found patients to be more satisfied with care provided by nurse practitioners than care provided by GPs. NHS Direct (telephone triage by nurses) has been found to be as effective as doctors in assessing whether patients need to be seen by a GP (Lattimer *et al.* 2000). This service has also been found to produce high patient satisfaction and to have a useful role in providing 'reassurance' to callers (O'Cathain *et al.* 2000).

The other distinctions between advanced nursing and medicine are the improved consistency, continuity and coordination of care that advanced nursing roles provide, aspects of care which are very difficult to deliver when care is otherwise provided by junior doctors who are rarely in post more than a few months. Preston *et al.* (1999) found that a lack of consistency across settings was a frequent source of problems and impeded patients' progress. It also produced feelings of anxiety and of not being valued as an individual. Continuity was achieved when a patient received care from a particular professional throughout the care process, and received constant coordinated care from different staff working together. Armstrong *et al.* (2002) found the ability of advanced nurse practitioners to provide continuity and coordination of care was seen as the principal benefit of these roles to patient care. Such nurses can act as a focal point for liaison and promote closer working relationships within the hospital and across care boundaries.

Undoubtedly, future research needs to address several unresolved issues in relation to advanced nursing practice and the distinctions and similarities with regard to medical roles. First, if patients are more satisfied with the care provided by advanced nurse practitioners, then factors that lead to this effect need to be further elucidated. Satisfaction with care could be related to many different factors. For instance, differences in the training and the consultation skills of nurses, patients' expectations, or the length of time such nurses spend in consultations.

Collaboration not confrontation in practice

Key to the success of advanced nursing roles is collaborative relationships with other members of the healthcare team. The idea of collaborative practice is fostered by government policy (DoH 1999a,b; NHS Executive 1999), with each of these documents including collaboration as an integral component of care. For the advanced nurse practitioner, a collaborative relationship with medical colleagues is particularly important. Advanced nursing roles disturb the traditional pattern of doctor–patient and doctor–nurse interaction as power relations and role boundaries shift, but a collaborative partnership helps to maintain the equilibrium.

Henneman *et al.* (1995) state that a relationship between individuals involved in collaboration is non-hierarchical. Power is shared and is based on knowledge and expertise rather than role or title. The concept of collaborative practice between nursing and medicine is widely written about, although it is difficult to find an agreed statement of meaning. Taylor perhaps offers one of the best definitions, stating that

> Collaborative practice incorporates a recognition of, and respect for, each participant's unique expertise in healthcare delivery. Doctors and nurses work together in a non-

hierarchical relationship, and both professionals contribute to decisions made together about patients. The relationship is characterised by trust and mutual communication. This leads to increased job satisfaction and better patient outcomes. (Taylor 1996: 69)

Collaboration also requires an environment with a team orientation (Evans & Carlson 1992), and an organisational structure that is flat rather than hierarchical (Henneman *et al.* 1995). Collaboration will substantiate the unique and important contribution made by individuals, reinforcing feelings of competence, self-worth and importance, and thereby promoting interprofessional cohesiveness (Henneman *et al.* 1995). Miccolo and Spanier (1993) highlight the role that collaboration plays in enhancing collegiality and respect among professionals. By forming a collaborative team, doctors and nurses can avoid turf battles and focus on the delivery of care. Strategies that address territorialism include focusing on the specific roles of each profession, along with corresponding education regarding the advanced nurse practitioner's responsibilities and clinical contributions. An ongoing environment of collaboration will be facilitated if there is a clear definition as to which patients are appropriate for each discipline, with consultation on a regular and consistent basis.

Many antecedents to collaboration are dependent on the readiness of individuals to engage in the aforementioned interpersonal processes. Readiness to engage in these processes will be affected by factors such as educational preparation, maturity, and prior experience of working in similar situations. Individuals need to have a clear understanding and acceptance of their own role, level of expertise and boundaries of practice. Good communication skills play a pivotal role in the promotion of collaboration. Effective communication requires that members of the team listen to each other's perspective, and yet be assertive in presenting their point of view relating to the process of care. Respect for, and recognition of, each professional's knowledge and judgement is a prerequisite to collaboration, and respect requires a basic level of understanding and acceptance of the expertise and roles of other professions. Trust is also an essential element for collaboration to flourish. A lack of trust presents an insurmountable barrier to the development of collaborative practice.

Henneman *et al.* (1995) suggest that a lack of collaborative practice may play a central role in the fragmentation of care, patient dissatisfaction and poor outcomes. Additionally, they claim that non-collaborative work environments may contribute to the role dissatisfaction routinely described by healthcare professionals. Collaborative practice does not have to equate to losing professional identity or values. It is possible to pursue a strategy collectively with shared initiatives, whilst also pursuing individual professional objectives. An obsession with the uniqueness of nursing as a profession can fail to recognise the synergy that results when professions with varying perspectives work together.

Collaborative practice is seen within the clinical setting when medical staff and advanced nurse practitioners work together as a team. The nurse functions independently and autonomously but there is the opportunity for frequent sharing of ideas and knowledge regarding patient care. In complex cases there will be discussion and exchange of ideas with a mutually agreeable decision. Sometimes the doctor will provide more insight and experience with respect to a particular problem and at other times the nurse has greater expertise. Such interprofessional collaboration brings together the skills and talents of both professions and creates an enhanced environment for better health outcomes that ultimately can translate to improved quality of care, quality of life and cost-effectiveness in healthcare delivery. Mundinger (1994) suggests that collaborative practice between the two professions is more effective and comprehensive than independent practice.

A view of advanced nursing from a medical perspective

Consultants and GPs should understand that advanced nursing practice might bring significant advantages to patient care, that the nurses in question are not doctor replacements and that they are complementary to a medical team. Many senior doctors have this understanding and share a vision of the future that has been elaborated above. However, as in any profession, there are always a few sceptics and 'dinosaurs', usually expressing sentiments such as 'doctoring on the cheap'. It is therefore essential that the advanced nurse practitioner receives proper training and adequate support.

The support must be at a personal, a clinical and a managerial level. The advanced nurse practitioner must be an integrated member of the team, not just an accessory. Clinical support is essential so that the nurse always has someone to liaise with on matters outside his or her boundaries of practice. At a managerial level the clinician must be prepared to share the responsibility for the day-to-day logistics of implementing new practices, the setting up of clinics, preparing protocols and information sheets, and generally making ready the infrastructure for a new member of the team. Hospital or primary care trusts must be appraised of the implementation of new advanced roles, as they will carry liability for the care delivered by the nurse. Public relations are important; prior notification of the implementation of new services is an essential component of success. Confirmation of the acceptability of a nurse undertaking advanced practice by questionnaire survey or audit will give the nurse the confidence that all is well and also serve to convince managers and colleagues that the process is valued and effective (Gidlow *et al.* 1997).

As a consultant who has worked with nurse practitioners for several years I know the extent to which advanced nursing practice has improved the working of a department. Efficiency and clinical risk have improved substantially. This is in no small part due to the continuity and diligence afforded by permanent fully trained members of staff and their approach to patient care; a style of care that is notably different from that of a doctor. The continuity of care is a feature about which patients most often express their appreciation. The same patient may well see the nurse in the clinic, then some time later on the ward before and after their surgery, and later again in the day unit for chemotherapy or cystoscopy.

It is important to put to one side the historical divide between doctors and nurses. I now see advanced nurse practitioners as being fully integrated into the clinical team. Our common vision is the delivery of high-quality care safely, efficiently and courteously. Tempting though it may be for some, it is inappropriate to attempt to equate a nurse practitioner with any given level of seniority within the medical hierarchy. Their knowledge and understanding, albeit within certain boundaries, is often much better than many doctors. Furthermore, their skill at minor surgical procedures can equate to those of a consultant (Gidlow *et al.* 2000).

The critical difference between the doctor and the nurse practitioner is that doctors, at all levels, are expected to work within their sphere of competence but that it is they themselves who are often left to define the boundaries of that competence. Nurses, on the other hand, by virtue of the fact that they do not have full medical training, must have those boundaries defined for them. They must be able to satisfy everyone concerned that they have the skills and training to discharge clinical care within those boundaries and recognise when there are clinical problems outside their scope and training. Thus it is those specialities that have many 'set piece' clinical scenarios that stand to benefit most from the nurse practitioner. Urology is such a speciality. Table 13.1 shows the wide spectrum of work undertaken by nurse practitioners in the Department of Urology at Ashford Hospital. The value of advanced nursing practice in the shape of the clinical nurse practitioner is beyond doubt. The challenge for the near future is to establish improved training and maintain adequate support for these nurses.

Table 13.1   Urology nurse practitioner duties within the Department of Urology, Ashford Hospital

Office	Ward
• Education and training PRHOs, SHOs, and ward staff	• Continuity
• Lecturing on advanced nursing practice	• Patient information
• Responsible for cancer data	• Scan bladders
• Surveillance of biopsy results	• Implement protocols
• Telephone follow-up	• Manage and supervise care pathways
• Run MDT cancer meetings	
• Advise community nurses and GPs	
• Research	
Day Unit	**Outpatient Dept**
• Intravesical chemotherapy	• BPH assessment clinic
• Trial of catheter removal	• Prostate cancer follow-up clinic
• Train patients in intermittent self-catheterisation	• Erectile dysfunction clinic
• Cystoscopy	• Urodynamics clinic
	• Outreach clinics in primary care

How to further good working practices

- *Provide a clear definition of the scope and purpose of advanced nursing roles.* The purpose of all advanced nursing roles should be to improve patient care. Such roles should not be seen simply as a means to fill the gaps left following the reduction in junior doctor availability. The goals and purpose of the role have to be clear in order for all staff to have a shared understanding of the role, and thus make it more likely to succeed.

- *Obtain support from senior medical and nursing staff and management before attempting to develop advanced nursing roles*. Introducing such roles is made much easier if local opinion leaders, such as senior consultants, lead GPs and senior nurses give their full support. Middle management also needs to support the role if it is to be effective. These are key persons to target before the development and implementation of such roles.

- *Involve other healthcare professionals and organisations in developing advanced nursing roles*. Whether the role is based in primary or secondary care, other healthcare professionals, such as radiologists, pharmacists, community nurses and GPs, have to be involved in developing the post. Other organisations, for example, primary care trusts, must also be involved if the role is to be successful and there is to be good cooperation between primary and secondary care. All healthcare professionals working with the advanced nurse practitioner need to clearly understand and agree where the boundaries of practice lie.

- *Education of other healthcare professionals and the public regarding advanced nursing roles*. Concise and informative literature needs to be provided to both patients and staff regarding the advanced nurse practitioner's scope of practice and clinical contributions. It is helpful if the information is presented in a manner that shows the complementary nature of collaborative practice between the disciplines and between medicine and nursing in particular. Patients and their families need to know the difference between advanced nurse practitioners and doctors. Nurses need to be aware of the legal implications of patients assuming they are doctors (Dowling *et al.* 1996). For these reasons advanced nursing roles need to be publicised more widely.

- *Education and training*. If nurses are to expand their role beyond traditional boundaries, important issues regarding training must be addressed. Inadequate in-house training programmes of a few days' duration are not sufficient. In-house training is not uniform and provides limited opportunities for professional development. The standardisation of competence through an accredited formal education programme will help to ensure safe practice and minimise risk to patients. Unfortunately, very few of such programmes are available in many specialities. Advanced nurse practitioners need to be active in lobbying for such courses to be more readily available. Until these accredited courses are established, it is incumbent on the nurse and the supervising medical practitioners to determine the level of knowledge and skill required to underpin the role. A structured training programme has to be developed with the nurse receiving core training and education against specified competences and knowledge.

- *Close collaboration with medical colleagues*. Nurses in advanced roles need to ensure that there are regular and consistent sessions for consultation with medical colleagues. This is best accomplished by regular scheduled meetings in which patient management and the scope of practice are discussed. Such meetings give opportunities for the nurse to highlight the benefits of their role with regard to patient education, family assessment and support, and community awareness. Collaborative working is enhanced if medical colleagues are readily accessible where nurse-led services are provided.

- *Role evaluation*. Robust role evaluation strategies must be developed to measure the effects on clinical outcomes, patient satisfaction and other aspects of healthcare, such as job satisfaction, effects on other healthcare professionals and costs. Outcomes need to be publicised as this will go some way to raising the awareness of such roles and reducing resistance.

Conclusion

Reforms in the NHS are bringing about a reduced reliance on medicine and an opportunity for nurses to have a more autonomous role in healthcare provision. There is currently a much greater emphasis on teamwork and collaborative practice with recognition that optimum patient care requires the insight of both doctors and nurses working independently. Studies have shown that patients appreciate the approach to care that advanced nurse practitioners provide, with high levels of patient satisfaction. The care provided by such nurses has been shown to be effective. Advanced nursing roles also improve the consistency, continuity and coordination of patient care. Collaborative relationships with medical colleagues are key to the success of advanced nursing roles. There has to be recognition and respect for each participant's unique expertise in healthcare delivery. The professions need to work together in a non-hierarchical relationship, both contributing to decisions made together about patients. The advanced nurse practitioner functions independently and autonomously but there is the opportunity for frequent sharing of ideas and knowledge regarding patient care. Such collaborative practice results in improved quality of care for patients.

  Key questions for Chapter 13

In your field of practice:

(1) How could the suggestions for good working practice be applied?
(2) What plans would you make to evaluate their effectiveness?
(3) In what ways might the interface between advanced practice and medicine be further researched?

References

Alcolado, J. (2000) Nurse practitioners and the future of general practice. *British Medical Journal*, 320: 1084.

Armstrong, S., Tolson, D. & West, B. (2002) Role development in acute nursing in Scotland. *Nursing Standard*, 16 (17): 33–8.

Barton, T., Thorne, R. & Hoptroff, M. (1999) The nurse practitioner: redefining occupational boundaries? *International Journal Nursing Studies*, 36: 57–63.

Centre for Health Services Research (1998) *Evaluation of Nurse Practitioners in General Practice in Northumberland: the EROS projects 1 & 2.* CHSR: University of Newcastle upon Tyne.

DoH (1997) *The New NHS: Modern, Dependable.* London: DoH.

DoH (1998) *Our Healthier Nation: A Contract for Health.* London: The Stationery Office.

DoH (1999a) *Making a Difference: Strengthening the Nursing, Midwifery and Health Visiting Contribution to Health and Healthcare.* London: DoH.

DoH (1996b) *Saving Lives: Our Healthier Nation.* London: DoH.

DoH (2000a). *The NHS Plan: A Plan for Investment, A Plan for Reform.* Wetherby: DoH.

DoH (2000b) *The NHS Cancer Plan: A Plan for Investment, A Plan for Reform.* Leeds: DoH.

Dowling, S., Martin, R., Skidmore, P., Doyal, L., Cameron, A. & Lloyd, S. (1996) Nurses taking on junior doctors' work: a confusion of accountability. *British Medical Journal*, 312: 1211–14.

English, T. (1997) Medicine in the 1990's needs a team approach. *British Medical Journal*, 314: 661–3.

Evans, S. & Carlson, R. (1992) Nurse/physician collaboration: solving the nursing shortage crisis. *American Journal of Critical Care*, 1 (1): 25–32.

Gidlow, A.B., Laniado, M.E., Kulkarni, R.P. & Ellis, B.W. (1997) Acceptability of a urology nurse practitioner by patients and their general practitioners. *British Journal of Urology*, 79 (Suppl. 4): 37.

Gidlow, A.B., Laniado, M.E. & Ellis, B.W. (2000) The nurse cystoscopist: a feasible option? *British Journal of Urology*, 85 (6): 651–4.

Henneman, E., Lee, J. & Cohen, J. (1995) Collaboration: a concept analysis. *Journal of Advanced Nursing*, 21: 103–9.

Henry, B. (1994) Rethinking nursing and medicine. *Image*, 26 (4): 254.

Horrocks, S., Anderson, E. & Salisbury, C. (2002) Systematic review of whether nurse practitioners working in primary care can provide equivalent care to doctors. *British Medical Journal*, 324: 819–23.

Hunsberger, M., Mitchell, A., Blatz, S. *et al.* (1992) Definition of an advanced practice role in the NICU: the clinical nurse specialist/neonatal practitioner. *Clinical Nurse Specialist*, 6 (2): 91–6.

Inui, T. (1994) Why doctors? *The Economist*, 333(7893): 117–18.

Kinnersley, P., Anderson, E., Parry, K. *et al.* (2000) Randomised controlled trial of nurse practitioner versus general practitioner care for patients requiring 'same day' consultations in primary care. *British Medical Journal*, 320: 1043–8.

Lattimer, V., Sassi, F., George, S. *et al.* (2000) Cost analysis of nurse telephone consultations in out of hours primary care: evidence from a randomised controlled trial. *British Medical Journal*, 320: 1053–7.

Miccolo, M. & Spanier, A. (1993) Critical care management in the 1990s: making collaborative practice work. *Critical Care Clinics*, 9 (3): 443–53.

Mundinger, M. (1994) Advanced practice nursing: good medicine for physicians? *New England Journal of Medicine*, 330 (4): 211–14.

NHS Executive (1996) *Nurse Practitioner Evaluation Project: Final Report.* Uxbridge: Coopers & Lybrand.

NHS Executive (1999) *Clinical Governance: Quality in the NHS.* London: NHS Executive.

O'Cathain, A., Munro, J., Nicholl, J. & Knowles, E. (2000) How helpful is NHS Direct? Postal survey of callers. *British Medical Journal*, 320: 1035.

Pearson, P. (1996) Are nurse practitioners merely substitute doctors? *Professional Nurse*, 11 (5): 325.

Preston, C., Cheater, F., Baker, R. & Hearnshaw, H. (1999) Left in limbo: patients' views on care across the primary/secondary interface. *Quality in Healthcare*, 8: 16–21.

Reveley, S. (1998) The role of the triage nurse practitioner in general medical practice: an analysis of the role. *Journal of Advanced Nursing*, 28: 584–91.

Reveley, S. (1999a) Development of the nurse practitioner role. In: *Nurse Practitioners Clinical Skills and Professional Issues* (eds M. Walsh, A. Crumbie & S. Reveley). Oxford: Butterworth-Heinemann.

Reveley, S. (1999b) Working with others: the nurse practitioner and role boundaries in primary healthcare. In: *Nurse Practitioners Clinical Skills and Professional Issues* (eds M. Walsh, A. Crumbie & S. Reveley). Oxford: Butterworth-Heinemann.

Reveley, S. & Haigh, K. (2001) Introducing the nurse practitioner role in a surgical unit: one nurse's journey. In: *Nurse Practitioners Clinical Skills and Professional Issues* (eds M. Walsh, A. Crumbie & S. Reveley). Oxford: Butterworth-Heinemann.

Reveley, S., Walsh, M. & Crumbie, A. (2001) Conclusions. In: *Nurse Practitioners Clinical Skills and Professional Issues* (eds M. Walsh, A. Crumbie & S. Reveley). Oxford: Butterworth-Heinemann.

Richardson, G. & Maynard, A. (1995) *Fewer Doctors? More Nurses? A Review of the Knowledge Base of Doctor–Nurse Substitution.* Discussion Paper 135. York: NHS Centre for Reviews & Dissemination, York Centre for Health Economics.

Royal College of Physicians (2000) *Hospital Doctors under Pressure: New Roles for the Healthcare Workforce.* London: Royal College of Physicians.

Shum, C., Humphreys, A., Wheeler, D. *et al.* (2000) Nurse management of patients with minor illnesses in general practice: multicentre randomised controlled trial. *British Medical Journal,* 320: 1038–43.

Stein, I., Watts, D. & Howell, T. (1990) The doctor–nurse game revisited. *New England Journal of Medicine,* 322 (8): 546–9.

Strauss, A., Fagerhaugh, S., Suczek, B. & Wiener, C. (1985) *Social Organisation of Medical Work.* Chicago: University of Chicago Press.

Taylor, J. (1996) Collaborative practice within the intensive care unit: a deconstruction. *Intensive Critical Care Nursing,* 12: 64–70.

UKCC (1992) *The Scope of Professional Practice.* London: UKCC.

Walsh, M. (2001) The nurse practitioner role in hospital: professional and organisational issues. In: *Nurse Practitioners Clinical Skills and Professional Issues* (eds M. Walsh, A. Crumbie & S. Reveley). Oxford: Butterworth-Heinemann.

Williams, S. (1998) Quality and care: patients' perceptions. *Nursing Care Quality,* 12 (6): 18–25.

Chapter 14

Nurse Prescribing and Advanced Practice

Peter Matthews

Introduction

The definition of advanced practice launched by the International Council of Nurses (ICN) makes clear that, as part of the move to increase access to health services, practitioners should be recognised as having the ability to act as the first, or in some instances, the only point of contact with health services (ICN 2002; see also WHO 2000). Inherent in this recognition is the authority to diagnose and prescribe treatment that includes medication. In the USA the authority of advanced practitioners to diagnose and prescribe is well-established and each state allows some form of prescribing authority (Pearson 2001). The gradual introduction and acceptance of prescribing rights indicates that advanced nurses are able to take responsibility for prescribing and to practise safely in this context.

This chapter presents a discussion of nurse prescribing in the UK. It begins with an account of the historical context in which proposals for the extension of prescribing rights to nurses has been examined and tested over a number of years. This is followed by a discussion of the contribution that nurses can make to care if they are able to prescribe and an explanation of the three situations in which they may now do so, namely as independent or supplementary prescribers or as part of patient group directions. The chapter then addresses issues in prescribing that include the preparation of practitioners, the principles of prescribing and the legal dimensions of the prescriber's role. The chapter closes by considering the future for advanced practitioners as prescribers and presents some key questions for further discussion.

The context of nurse prescribing

The origin of the present empowerment of nurses to prescribe medicines within the NHS is contained in the report of Baroness Cumberledge, published in 1986, on the future of community nursing. The report identified improvements in patient care and efficiency that would arise from community nurses being allowed to prescribe dressings and wound care products for their patients. The review recommended that the Department of Health and Social Security (DHSS), later split and renamed the Department of Health (DoH) and the Department of Work and Pensions (DWP), should agree a limited list of items and simple agents that may be prescribed by nurses and issue guidance to enable nurses to control drug dosage in well-defined circumstances. Following on from this the Advisory Group on Nurse Prescribing chaired by Dr June Crown made detailed proposals for the introduction of prescribing by selected nurses. This report recommended a Nurse's Formulary and identified the training, funding and legislative changes that would be required. It also recommended swift action to implement nurse prescribing by 1 April 1992 following an evaluation study to identify views of patients, relatives and healthcare professionals and a full economic appraisal.

Despite the enthusiasm and urgency identified by the Advisory Group, it was not until 1994 that the first nurse prescribing demonstration sites were established based on eight fundholding practices, and two years later Bolton Community Health NHS Trust implemented nurse prescribing on a community basis. Fundholding was a concept introduced by the National Health Service and Community Care Act 1990 within which GPs had a greater involvement in the control of practice budgets, including prescribing budgets. Using their budgetary freedoms, such practices often led the way in exploring innovative ways of delivering improved healthcare. Fundholding ended in 1999 (Health Act 1999 c.8). By 1997 nurse-prescribing projects had been established in all NHS regions in England. These pilots were successful and showed that nurse prescribing produced better targeted prescribing of wound management products and more cost-effective prescribing of items such as arm slings, bandages and dressings. In addition it reduced workload for GPs, improved patient convenience and enhanced the job satisfaction/professional responsibility for the nurses involved. It was agreed that nurse prescribing should be extended throughout England, and Health Circulars (DoH 1998a, 1999a) defining the processes to be followed. The NHS Plan identified an expanded role for nurses, and included in the Chief Nursing Officer for Englands 10 key roles for nurses was the prescribing of medicines and treatments (DoH 2000a). By September 2001, more than 22 000 district nurses and health visitors, including around 1000 practice nurses who held one of these qualifications, had been trained to prescribe. The range of medicines that they were authorised to prescribe was defined by the Nurse Prescribers' Formulary and were required to be included in the *Drug Tariff*.[1]

Whilst these developments were taking place the DoH set up in March 1997 under the leadership of Dr June Crown a group to review the prescribing, supply and administration of medicines. The first report of this group was published in April 1998 and made recommendations on the supply and administration of medicines by group protocols (DoH 1998b). This had been considered as an urgent matter since many nurses employed in hospitals were giving prescription-only medicines (POMs) routinely within nursing guidelines. The guidelines were often of variable quality and usually of doubtful legal status. The review recommended that the majority of patients should receive medication on an individually prescribed basis but recognised that in some situations it was advantageous to the patient for nurses to be able to administer medication without a prescription and that this should be under a group protocol. The report established criteria for the content and process of developing group protocols and recommended clarification of the laws relating to the supply of medicines under group protocols.

The necessary changes to the Medicines Act 1968 were made in a series of amendment orders that came into force on 9 August 2000 and the process for developing group protocols, now called patient group directions (PGDs), was established within the NHS on the same date (DoH 2000b). The Royal Pharmaceutical Society of Great Britain has published a useful detailed description of PGDs.[2]

The final Crown report was published in March 1999 and recommended extending the legal authority to prescribe medicines within the NHS to groups of healthcare professionals beyond the existing medical and dental practitioners (DoH 1999b). It recommended that the legal authority to prescribe should be linked to competence and expertise and that prescription-only medicines (POMs) should be included. The report introduced the concept of independent and dependent (subsequently changed to supplementary) prescribers, and introduced working definitions of the two roles. The report also made recommendations on training, monitoring and the mechanisms for recognising new groups of prescribers. Throughout the report's recommendations, patient safety and benefit were paramount in the extension of prescribing rights.

In May 2001, the Health Minister, Lord Philip Hunt, announced the government's intention to have 10 000 independent nurse prescribers, now known as extended nurse prescribers, by 2004. This was accompanied by the allocation of £10 million to support the training programme. Unlike the earlier programme, which envisaged that almost all nurses within the eligible groups would become prescribers, the independent prescribers would be selected by employing authorities in consultation with local healthcare practitioners in the light of local priorities. Criteria to be used in the selection of candidates for the training programme included an assessment that they were capable of study at first degree level, had at least three years' post-qualification clinical experience and were in a post where they would have regular opportunity and

---

[1] Published monthly by The Stationery Office.
[2] Royal Pharmaceutical Society of Great Britain (2000) *Patient Group Directions: A Resource Pack for Pharmacists.* London: Royal Pharmaceutical Society, Professional Standards Directorate.

need to prescribe for patients within defined clinical categories. Employers of nurses selected for training as extended nurse prescribers were to give a commitment to providing time and facilities for appropriate continuing professional development and, very importantly, give access to a prescribing budget. The nurse was also required be legally eligible to prescribe. Eligibility was defined as:

- Being a First Level Registered Nurse or Midwife
- Having valid registration with the United Kingdom Central Council for Nursing, Midwifery and Health Visiting (UKCC)
- Successfully completing the nurse prescribing preparation and obtaining a mark to indicate this on the Register.

On successful completion of the training the nurse was required to undertake a mandatory period of prescribing supervised by a doctor. Once qualified, nurses would have greatly expanded prescribing rights enabling them to prescribe a wide range of POMs, including some antibiotics. Prescribing would be limited to the treatment of specified conditions, including minor injuries such as burns, cuts or sprains; minor ailments such as hay fever or ear infections; promoting healthier lifestyles such as providing vitamins for women planning pregnancy; and palliative care.

The intention was to improve patient access and remove work from over-pressured GPs and hospital doctors (DoH 2001). Expanding nurse prescribing was a key part of the government's strategy to modernise the NHS and make the most of its employees' skills and knowledge. Prescribing by nurses, pharmacists and others was a fundamental part of the NHS Plan and was also a reflection of international changes that showed benefits of economy and efficiency arising from the extension of prescribing rights. The changes empowered appropriately trained independent nurse prescribers to prescribe all general sales list and pharmacy medicines prescribable by doctors under the NHS, together with a list of POMs linked to the specified medical conditions mentioned earlier. By April 2002 the first extended nurse prescribers had completed their training and were registered to prescribe from a list of drugs contained within the Nurse Prescribers' Extended Formulary, published in the *Drug Tariff*, which included a range of POMs drawn up by the Medicines Control Agency (MCA) after wide consultation.

At the time of writing there are proposals for a further extension of prescribing rights, known as supplementary prescribing, for nurses and a range of healthcare practitioners, including pharmacists, to enable them to support the continuing care of patients following a clinical assessment and agreed treatment programme developed by an independent prescriber (MCA 2002).

Contribution of nurse prescribing to patient care

The reviews and legislative changes referred to earlier were driven and informed by a number of social and political realisations. The NHS of the 1950s was no longer acceptable to a society used to wide variety of choice, ease of access to other services and convenience coupled with quality. At a time of increased demand, arising from a combination of a growing elderly population, diminishing number of GPs and hospital doctors, continual development of drug technology and high public expectations, it was clear that changes needed to be made.

For many years, with the expanding role of nurses, it had been widespread practice for nurses in both primary and secondary care to make decisions on prescribing, but these had to be referred to the medical practitioner for a prescription to be issued. With the advent of nurse prescribing and extended nurse prescribing the nurse prescriber is now in a position to make a clinical evaluation of a patient, agree a treatment pathway with the patient, and write the prescription all in the course of a single consultation. The advantages of easy access, usually a longer period of consultation and speedy initiation of treatment are of great benefit to the patient (Venning *et al.* 2000). By reducing the need for a medical consultation and prescription-writing, the GPs time is freed up for more appropriate consultations and as a result patient access is increased by both nurses and doctors being able to prescribe. Recent changes in the delivery of primary care services have moved away from a GP-centred system to a team-based approach in which a range of healthcare professionals can interact directly with the patient in accordance with the patients clinical need and the practitioners own skills. Nurse prescribing not only enhances the nursing role within the team but also promotes a closer clinical relationship with the patient and improves adherence to treatment. Furthermore, nurse prescribing enables a full clinical service to be provided to parts of the community such as travellers, the homeless and asylum seekers who, because of their lifestyle, were previously disadvantaged in this respect.

The categories of prescriber/supplier

The new legislation has given rise to three situations in which medicines may be prescribed or supplied and it is important to be aware of the freedoms and limitations attached to each.

First, *patient group directions* involve a nurse who is authorised to supply or administer medicines, including POMs, to groups of patients who may not be individually identified before presentation for treatment. Patient group directions (PGDs) should be reserved for those limited situations where they offer an advantage for patient care without compromising patient safety and where they are consistent with appropriate professional relationships and accountability. The PGD must be signed by a doctor/dentist and a pharmacist and empowers the nurse to supply and/or administer medicines specified by the PGD to categories of patients defined within the PGD for the treatment of specified conditions. The empowerment is restricted to the number of doses that may be supplied and, where appropriate, the PGD will state exclusions that the nurse must adhere to.

PGDs have proved valuable in situations where a limited range of indications apply to a large number of patients. These situations require that the condition to be treated can be clearly defined and that the treatment to be administered is limited to a single medicine. A typical example in primary care is the use of PGDs to authorise a nurse to give vaccinations, whilst in secondary care the examples range from the provision of emergency hormonal contraception by family planning nurses through to the administration of muscle relaxants within intensive care units. It is important to distinguish between the acts of supplying/administering a medicine and prescribing a medicine. A PGD cannot authorise a nurse to prescribe medicine within the NHS.

Second, the *independent nurse prescriber* is a nurse authorised to make a clinical assessment, usually including a diagnosis, decide, in consultation with the patient, an appropriate treatment plan, and if prescribing is appropriate, write any necessary prescriptions for dispensing within the NHS. In this situation the patient may be presenting for the first time within an episode of care. Within the limits of their professional judgement, independent nurse prescribers have the freedom to change the medicine or alter the dose/frequency of administration at any time during the episode of care without reference to anyone else.

The group of independent nurse prescribers may be registered as district nurse/health visitor prescribers or extended formulary nurse prescribers. The distinctions between these categories are dealt with later in this chapter in the section on legal aspects. The range of conditions for which the nurse may prescribe is clearly defined and has been referred to earlier. It is certain that, as the experience of nurse prescribing grows, this list will be expanded. One can see many benefits in expanding nurse prescribing to cover mental health, diabetes, asthma, rheumatology and many other specialist areas in hospital and primary care practice. The range of medicines that may be prescribed is also defined and this list is printed in the *Drug Tariff* and as an appendix to the *British National Formulary* (BNF).[3]

Third, the *supplementary prescriber's* role in patient care begins once a diagnosis has been established and a written treatment plan has been agreed with an independent prescriber. In the consultation process on establishing supplementary prescribers it is envisaged that this independent prescriber must be either a doctor or a dentist. The independent prescriber may transfer responsibility for the continuing clinical management of the patient to the supplementary prescriber. The decision to transfer responsibility will be subject to agreement by both the patient and the supplementary prescriber. The treatment plan will specify the medicines that may be prescribed and the range of options that are available to the supplementary prescriber as well as define the necessary monitoring criteria. It is the intention that supplementary prescribers will be responsible for maintaining clinical care, including any prescribing requirements for patients with chronic illness. At the time of writing it is expected that legislation will be in place by 2003 to allow suitably trained nurses and pharmacists to take on the responsibilities of supplementary prescribers.

Supporting prescribing is the *Drug Tariff*, produced by the Prescription Pricing Authority (PPA) on behalf of the DoH and updated each month. It is the definitive list of those products that may be prescribed within the NHS at public expense. The *Tariff* is a guide to prescribers as to what they may prescribe and to pharmacists as to what they may dispense. In the case of dressings and appliances, pharmacists may dispense only the specific products described within the *Tariff*. The *Tariff* also lists those medicines that may not be prescribed within the NHS. Provision has been made for all nurse prescribers to receive copies of the *Drug Tariff* at six-monthly intervals. If a nurse

---

[3] Published by the British Medical Association and the Royal Pharmaceutical Society of Great Britain.

is prescribing a new product it would be prudent to check in the current month's *Tariff* that it is included. All GPs and pharmacists receive updated copies on a monthly basis.

Preparation for the prescribing role

Programmes of preparation for nurses, midwives and health visitors to prescribe from the Nurse Prescribers' Extended Formulary (NPEF) began in January 2002, after extensive work by the UKCC, DoH and the English National Board for Nursing, Midwifery and Health Visiting (ENB). The preparation consists of a taught component at degree level of 25 days in the university plus 12 nurse practice days when a designated medical practitioner provides the student with supervision, support and opportunities to develop competence in prescribing practice. The medical practitioner must be either an appropriately qualified GP or a hospital doctor above specialist registrar grade. The programme is part-time and spread over a period of three months. The purpose of this part of the training is to allow the nurse to become familiar with the consultation process and the interpersonal skills and questioning techniques involved. The development of a clinical management plan and the use of critical appraisal will also be practised during this period. The programme ends with an assessment of theory and competence in prescribing. Existing district nurse/health visitor prescribers are eligible for consideration for training.

Competence in prescribing

Defining competence is difficult. In its guide on maintaining prescribing competences, the National Prescribing Centre (NPC 2001) divided competences into task-based and behaviourally based concepts. The NPC guide uses a behaviourally based approach, breaks the prescribing process into three main blocks and, by the use of carefully developed statements, enables nurses to structure their reflections on their prescribing practice. The first section is concerned with the consultation and identifies the knowledge necessary for high-quality, safe prescribing. The section defines steps to ensure that a diagnosis is established, treatment option appraisal is undertaken and satisfactory follow-up occurs. Behaviours appropriate to effective communication with the patient are identified. The second section concentrates on effective prescribing and identifies knowledge, activities and behaviours designed to achieve the most effective and safe use of medicines. The final section gives guidance on information sources, medicines-use frameworks both nationally and locally, appropriate consideration of the use of scarce resources, and draws attention to the issues around team working, self-awareness and confidence.

Principles of prescribing

The decision to prescribe medication as a result of making a clinical diagnosis is, to paraphrase Winston Churchill, not the end of the consultation but the end of the beginning of the consultation. Prescribing should be a logical, deductive process that takes account of the diagnosis, the characteristics of the patient, the evidence supporting the use of the particular choice of medicine and a considered balance of the benefits and risks involved. Once this decision has been taken by the prescriber it is necessary for the patient to be fully engaged in taking the treatment correctly and for the necessary length of time if a successful clinical outcome is to be secured. This is of particular importance where the condition is chronic and essential if it is both chronic and asymptomatic. Achieving success from the prescribing of statins in patients with increased cardiovascular risk is a good example of the latter case. Studies have shown that possibly one-third of patients for whom statins are prescribed cease to take their medication after the first year (Mitka 2001). This represents a significant failure to achieve the clinical outcome of reducing the risk of a serious cardiovascular event, exposure of patients to potentially serious side-effects for no advantage, and enormous waste of money and time. It is vital that the prescriber secures a shared contract (concordance) with the patient as part of the prescribing process.

The stages involved in prescribing

Stage one should review the holistic needs of the patient and whether medication is an appropriate response. It is not uncommon for patients to present with symptoms of a simple illness whilst having major underlying problems. It is important to recognise this situation and not to rush into treating the obvious condition with a prescription. The first line of approach to many conditions may involve attempts at lifestyle changes before resorting to medication. The prescriber needs to be aware of this. Is the patient expecting a prescription? It is clear that many patients do not expect a prescription but seek a consultation for reasons such as reassurance or the elimination of the possibility of serious illness (Britten & Ukoumunne 1997; Cockburn & Pit 1997). Some patients will expect and pressurise prescribers for a prescription for a variety of personal reasons other than to gain treatment for their medical condition. A prescription may be used to legitimise the sick role in the eyes of employers or family members, or just to gain attention. After due consideration of all these factors the nurse prescriber must decide if they are competent to proceed or if the patient needs referral to a GP.

Stage two should identify the desired outcomes of the intervention. If it is an acute illness then symptomatic relief or complete resolution is an achievable outcome. For chronic conditions, symptomatic relief, slowing the rate of deterioration or only partial achievement of these objectives may be the only possible approaches.

Stage three is the choice of an appropriate medicine. Prescribers should attempt to construct a range of medicines based on good evidence of efficacy, safety and cost-effectiveness. Wherever possible the first choice should be made from this list. By choosing from a small list the prescriber may accumulate considerable experience in using the drugs, identifying side effects and predicting outcomes. If the medicine is not appropriate for the particular patient then an alternative medicine should be used. Possible reasons for not using the first choice might be side effects that would exacerbate a coexisting condition such as prescribing a betablocker for hypertension for a patient with asthma. The age of the patient might require a second-line drug to be used.

Stage four is discussion with the patient of the medication, possible side effects, duration of treatment and expected outcomes. The patient needs to be aware of why they are being prescribed the medication, the name of the medication, the dose that they are to take, how to take it, how long it will take to work and possible side effects. They should be informed of the action to be taken, if any, as a result of side effects. It is important that the prescriber communicates this information effectively since there is considerable evidence that patients do not retain much of the information given to them during the consultation.

Stage five should secure the patient's agreement to take the medication. There is evidence that patients with serious illnesses regularly default on medicine-taking. For some conditions this is acceptable, but for others it may result in total treatment failure or worse. In these situations it is vital that the patient understands and agrees to their part of the prescribing partnership.

Stage six is the writing of the prescription. This is dealt with in some detail in a later section.

Stage seven is to ensure that full records are made. It is essential that full, accurate and timely records are made of all consultations, whether or not a prescription is issued. Guidance on record-keeping by nurses is contained in the UKCC *Guidelines for Records and Recordkeeping* (UKCC 1998). When a prescription is issued the record should show the name of the medicine, the dose and frequency, the total quantity prescribed, the route of administration and the date. A record should be made of any explanations/cautions given to the patient. Any reasons for not issuing a prescription should be recorded. The patient's GP records should be amended as soon as possible after the prescription has been given and certainly within 48 hours. The GP record should include the name of the nurse prescriber and should show that it is a nurse prescription.

Stage eight is the monitoring of the patient's progress at regular intervals appropriate to the individual's condition and stage of treatment. If the patient is not responding in accordance with the expected outcomes it is necessary to consider that the patient is not taking the medicine or the one prescribed is not effective. This should lead to questions about side effects, lack of clinical effectiveness, and poor motivation by the patient. Answers to these questions may lead the prescriber to change the dose, formulation or medicine.

Stage nine is reflecting on the prescribing. Reflection on all aspects of the nurse's activities is an important element of good practice (UKCC 1992). Prescribing is part of an active cycle of events in the treatment of patients, and reflection on the process is an essential part of improving performance. Self-questioning around the effectiveness of the medicine, side-effect profile, speed of onset, patient acceptability and final outcome will lead to the increased use of effective interventions and the reduction of less useful treatments. Using the Prescription Analysis can assist in developing a personal formulary or evaluating the consistency of prescribing decisions and cost (PACT) reports available from the Prescription Pricing Authority.

Writing the prescription

Once the decision has been taken that a medicine or medicines are the appropriate response to the patient's clinical needs and a full discussion has taken place with the patient and their agreement to this course of action has been secured then the pre-scription should be written. The law (Statutory Instrument 1997 No. 1830 The Prescription Only Medicines (Human Use) Order 1997) requires that the prescription, if it is for a POM, shall

(1) Be signed in ink (or other indelible substance) with the name of the appropriate practitioner giving it. If it is an NHS prescription then a computer printed form is allowed
(2) Contain the following particulars:
    (a) the address of the prescriber
    (b) the date
    (c) such particulars as indicate whether the prescriber is a doctor, a dentist, an appropriate nurse practitioner, a veterinary surgeon or a veterinary practitioner
    (d) where the prescriber is a doctor, dentist or appropriate nurse practitioner, the name, address and the age, if under 12 years, of the person for whose treatment it is given although in practice it is recommended that the age/date of birth is always stated
(3) Not be dispensed after the end of the period of six months from the appropriate date, unless it is a repeatable prescription in which case it shall not be dispensed for the first time after the end of that period nor otherwise than in accordance with the directions contained in the repeatable prescription. In addition, in the case of a repeatable prescription which does not specify the number of times it may be dispensed, it shall not be dispensed on more than two occasions unless it is a prescription for an oral contraceptive in which case it may be dispensed six times before the end of the period of six months from the appropriate date.

For the purposes of prescribing within the NHS, it is required that these conditions are met for all prescriptions whether or not the medicine is a POM. At the time of writing, repeatable prescriptions are not allowed within the NHS; however, pilot sites are investigating the potential of such a system and early change is anticipated. Repeatable prescriptions are single prescription forms that may be dispensed by a pharmacist on more than one occasion as specified by the prescriber. Repeat prescriptions, however, are prescriptions that are issued at regular intervals (normally 28 days) for the treatment of chronic conditions, where the medicines and doses are identical from one prescription form to the next. They may be dispensed on only one occasion.

For prescriptions written within the NHS by appropriate nurse prescribers the only prescription form that may be used is the lilac-coloured form FP10P. These forms are printed either with the words 'District Nurse/Health Visitor Prescriber' or 'Extended Formulary Nurse Prescriber' as appropriate. The restrictions applying to the use of each form are detailed later in this chapter. Hospital-based nurse prescribers will normally have their prescriptions dispensed in the hospital pharmacy and will use the appropriate locally agreed form. If it is intended that the prescription be dispensed by a community pharmacist then the nurse should use the orange-coloured FP10HP prescription form. The nurse should stamp the form 'Extended Formulary Nurse Prescriber UKCC No.... [to be entered by the nurse]'.

The body of the prescription should contain:

(1) The name of the medicine. The approved (generic) name should be used unless the medicine contains several ingredients, is a modified release product where the BNF recommends using the proprietary (trade) name, or special circumstances exist where the prescriber feels it is essential to specify a particular product (usually a dressing or appliance).
(2) The form of the medicine. Tablet, capsule, syrup, etc.
(3) The strength of the medicine.
(4) The dose to be taken and the frequency. If the medicine is to be taken as required then a minimum dose interval should be specified.
(5) The amount to be dispensed. This is preferably indicated by the number of days to be supplied. As required medicines must be prescribed by quantity. Where more than one medicine is prescribed on the form it is important that the number of days' supply is the same for all. This reduces waste and improves convenience for nurse, patient and carers.

Full details of good practice in prescription writing can be found at the beginning of the *British National Formulary* (BNF).

Legal issues in prescribing

The law concerning the prescribing, supply and administration of medicinal products is to be found in the Medicines Act 1968 and subordinate legislation made under it. Medicines are grouped into three legal categories based on potency, risk of side effects and the need for supply to be professionally supervised. The categories are:

- General sales list medicines (GSL). These may be supplied from a wide range of business premises. The medicines may only be supplied in unopened manufacturers' packs.
- Pharmacy-only medicines (P). These may only be sold or supplied from registered pharmacy premises and the supply must be by or under the supervision of a pharmacist. Some limited exemptions to these requirements exist.
- Prescription-only medicines (POM). These may normally only be sold or supplied in accordance with a signed and dated prescription issued by an appropriate practitioner. The appropriate practitioner was originally a doctor or dentist.

The Medicinal Products: Prescriptions by Nurses etc. Act 1992 c.28 extended prescribing rights to 'registered nurses, midwives and health visitors who are of such a description and comply with such conditions as may be specified in the order'.

Section 41 of the 1977 NHS Act was amended by the 1992 Act to allow health authorities to arrange for prescribing services provided by nurses, and enabled pharmacists to be paid for dispensing prescriptions signed by nurse practitioners. The 1992 Act was implemented in 1994 (Statutory Instrument 1994 No. 2408 c.48 The Medicinal Products: Prescriptions by Nurses etc. Act 1992 (Commencement No. 1) Order 1994).

A nurse prescriber was originally defined as a person who

- Is registered on parts 1–12 of the UKCC register
- Has a district nurse qualification and is employed by a health authority, trust or fundholding practice
- Is registered on Part 11 as a health visitor and is employed by a health authority, trust or fundholding practice
- Is named on the Professional Register and marked as qualified to prescribe (Statutory Instrument 1994 No. 2402 The National Health Service (Pharmaceutical Services and Charges for Drugs and Appliances) Amendment Regulations 1994).

The term 'nurse prescriber' was changed in 1997 to become 'appropriate nurse practitioner'. This was again changed in 2002 to distinguish between nurses authorised to prescribe from the Nurse Prescribers' Formulary (NPF), now referred to as 'district nurse/health visitor prescriber' and nurses authorised to prescribe from the *Nurse Prescribers' Extended Formulary* (NPEF) called 'extended formulary nurse prescriber' (Statutory Instrument 2002 No. 549 Prescription Only Medicines (Human Use) Amendment Order 2000). An extended formulary nurse prescriber is defined as a person:

> who is registered in Parts 1, 3, 5, 8, 10, 11, 12, 13, 14 or 15 of the professional register; and against whose name is recorded in that register an annotation signifying that he is qualified to order drugs, medicines and appliances from the Extended Formulary.

The medicinal products which nurses can prescribe are listed either in the NPF for district nurses and health visitors or in the NPEF, published as appendices to the BNF and contained within the *Drug Tariff*. District nurse/health visitor prescribers are limited to prescribing only the products included in the NPF list, whereas extended formulary nurse prescribers are authorised to prescribe all licensed P and GSL medicines prescribable on the NHS (except controlled drugs) and any POM listed in the NPEF but only by the route or form specified in the NPEF. Neither category of prescriber may prescribe presentations or pack sizes that are excluded from prescription under the NHS (Schedule 10 of the National Health Service (General Medical Services) Regulations 1992); these are listed in part XVIIIA of the *Drug Tariff*.

In addition to the legal aspects concerning the control of medicines the nurse prescriber has a number of other legal issues to contend with. The person signing a prescription is legally responsible for the consequences of that action, and in a society increasingly inclined to seek financial compensation for any untoward event the nurse prescriber must ensure that their role and range of duties are fully agreed with their employers before undertaking any prescribing. The duty of care owed to the patient by the nurse prescriber requires, among other things, that the nurse is adequately trained and prepared for prescribing, is aware of and works within the standards of care expected for safe prescribing, and abides by appropriate professional standards. A significant element of the duty of care is participation in continuing professional development and the maintenance of prescribing competences. Full guidance on these aspects is contained within the Nursing and Midwifery Council Code of Professional Conduct (NMC 2002).

The NHS spends around £4 billion on medicines each year, most of which is accounted for by prescribed medicines. With such a vast amount of money involved, prescription-related fraud exists. Regrettably, a small number of healthcare practitioners become involved in some aspect of this fraud and it is important for the nurse prescriber to be aware of good practice. Theft of prescription forms gives access to medication that may be sold or abused. Nurse prescribers must ensure that prescription forms are stored securely and that no one is allowed to borrow or use their forms. Prescribers need to be aware of patients who are using deceit to obtain unnecessary medicines for whatever purpose, and in these circumstances they should refuse to issue a prescription. Prescribing for patients that have not been clinically assessed by the prescriber in response to requests from non-prescribing colleagues may expose the prescriber to a range of clinical or probity-based complaints and it should not be undertaken without serious consideration of the possible consequences.

Conclusion

For many years prescribing was solely the province of the GP, and the establishment of effective relationships between nurse prescribers, GPs and, in the future, a range of other practitioners with prescribing rights, will take time to develop. In the interests of safety, speedy communication of prescribing actions and recording in a central GP-based patient record is essential. This will be assisted with the rapid development of electronic communication within the NHS. Of particular value will be the creation of a centralised electronic health record (EHR) and a locally based electronic patient record (EPR) that will be accessible to all practitioners with a valid need to do so. Pilot sites to develop this were operational in 2001 and it is planned that these services will be fully available, together with the electronic transmission of prescriptions from prescriber to pharmacist, by 2008 (DoH 2002). The EHR and EPR will not replace the need for face-to-face contact with all members of the team looking after a patient in order to establish an overall philosophy of care. Electronic systems will speed up communication, reduce the possibility of prescribing error and enable the pooling of the team's clinical wisdom directed at the treatment of individual patients.

The nurse prescriber will require support in assimilating new developments in medicines, and pharmacist colleagues in hospital and primary care will provide that support and also a ready access to medicines information. The pharmacist is able to provide assistance in enabling patients to take their medication regularly and can be a useful source of advice as to the difficulties that individual patients may be experiencing with their medicines.

Early experiences of nurse prescribing in the USA highlighted the advantages to patients and to healthcare delivery systems, and this led to rapid expansion of the range of prescribable medicines and the therapeutic areas in which nurse prescribers were authorised to work. From small beginnings, legislation is in place today in all states to allow nurse prescribing, although considerable variation in detail exists. Across the world a number of countries are in the process of implementing legislation to allow nurse prescribing, recognising its contribution to improved patient care, set against a background of increased levels of morbidity and reduced access to traditional models of medical-practitioner-delivered care. It is clear that prescribing is becoming an increasingly important element of the advanced nurse practitioner's portfolio of skills and further developments will contribute significantly to improved patient care.

? **Key questions for Chapter 14**

In your field of practice:

(1) In what ways could prescribing enhance patient care delivered by an advanced practitioner?
(2) How could patients' views on and satisfaction with nurse prescribing be assessed?
(3) How could the authority to prescribe enhance interdisciplinary collaboration?

References

Britten, N. & Ukoumunne, O. (1997) The influence of patients' hopes of receiving a prescription on doctor's perceptions and the decision to prescribe: a questionnaire survey. *British Medical Journal*, 315: 1506–10.

Cockburn, J. & Pit, S. (1997) Prescribing behaviour in clinical practice: patients' expectations and doctors' perceptions of patients' expectations – a questionnaire study. *British Medical Journal*, 315: 520–3.

DoH (1998a) *Nurse Prescribing: Implementing the Scheme Across England*, Health Service Circular 1998/232.

DoH (1998b) *Review of Prescribing, Supply and Administration of Medicines: A Report on the Supply and Administration of Medicines under Group Protocols*. London: DoH.

DoH (1999a) *Nurse Prescribing: Notification Details for Practice Nurse Prescribers*, Health Service Circular 1999/045.

DoH (1999b) *Review of Prescribing, Supply and Administration of Medicines: A Report on the Supply and Administration of Medicines under Group Protocols. Final report*. London: DoH.

DoH (2000a) *The NHS Plan: A Plan for Investment, A Plan for Reform*. Wetherby: DoH.

DoH (2000b) *Patient Group Directions (England Only)*, Health Service Circular 2000/026.

DoH (2001) Press release 2001/0223. London: DoH.

DoH (2002) *Delivering 21st Century IT Support for the NHS: National Strategic Programme*. London: DoH.

ICN (2002) http://icn.org (accessed September 2002).

MCA (2002) *Proposals for Supplementary Prescribing by Nurses and Pharmacists and Proposed Amendments to the Prescription Only Medicines (Human Use) Order 1997 MLX 284*, London: MCA.

Mitka, M. (2001) Cardiologists like statins – more than patients do. *Journal of the American Medical Association*, 286: 279–800.

NMC (2002) *Code of Professional Conduct*. London: NMC.

NPC (2001) *Maintaining competency in prescribing*. Liverpool: NPC.

Pearson, L. (2001) Annual legislative update. How each state stands on legislative issues affecting advanced nursing practice. *The Nurse Practitioner*, 26 (1): 7, 11–15, 17–18, 21–7, 28, 31–8, 47–54, 57.

UKCC (1992) *The Scope of Professional Practice*. London: UKCC.

UKCC (1998) *Guidelines for Records and Record Keeping*. London: UKCC.

Venning, P., Durie, A., Roland, M., Roberts, C. & Leese, B. (2000) Randomised controlled trial comparing cost effectiveness of general practitioners and nurse practitioners in primary care. *British Medical Journal*, 320: 1048–53.

WHO (2000) *Global Advisory Group on Nursing and Midwifery. Report of the 6th Meeting*. Geneva: WHO, Available at www.who.org (accessed September 2002).

Chapter 15

Legal and Ethical Issues in Advanced Practice

Bridgit Dimond

Introduction

The legal and ethical issues arising in advanced practice are so numerous and complex that they could justify a book in their own right. However, the aim of this chapter is to provide a general introduction to the legal context within which the advanced practitioner works and then explore in detail some of the more relevant issues. In place of the key questions, a list of recommended reading about legal issues is provided to facilitate further examination of this aspect of advanced practice.

Basic legal principles

The law in the UK arises from two main sources: Acts of Parliament or directives and regulations of the European Community – known as statute law; and the common law or judge-made law or case law which are the rulings laid down in the courts of this country or by the European Court of Justice (the court of the European Community) or by the European Court of Human Rights in Strasbourg.

Statute law

The process of creating legislation in this country usually starts with a Green Paper issued for consultation by a government department, which, following feedback, leads to the publication of a White Paper which sets out government policy. Following the White Paper, a bill is introduced into Parliament and goes through several readings in the House of Commons and House of Lords. When finally amended and approved by them the bill receives Royal Assent and becomes an Act. The Act does not necessarily come into force on being signed by the Queen, but dates for the different sections coming into force may be set out in statutory instruments (secondary legislation) that are laid before the Houses of Parliament for approval. Following devolution, the Assemblies of Scotland, Northern Ireland and Wales have varying law-making powers.

Common law

Inevitably, statutes and statutory instruments have to be interpreted. Where legal conflicts arise, judges are asked to interpret legislation and apply the law to a specific situation. Thus legal principles are set down, and the doctrine of precedent requires the lower courts to follow the principles laid down by higher courts. The House of Lords, as the most senior court, is alone able to decide not to follow its own decisions.

The courts do not have the power to overrule a statute, although the judges could comment adversely upon it. Where there are no statutes to cover a specific situation, then judges have to create law to fill the vacuum until such time as Parliament passes appropriate legislation. This is the present situation in relation to decision-making on behalf of mentally incapacitated adults. In the UK (apart from Scotland which has the Adult Incapacity (Scotland) Act 2000), when health professionals are caring for mentally incapacitated adults, they act under powers recognised by the House of

Lords in the case of *Re. F. v. West Berkshire Health Authority* (1989) 2 All ER 545. The unsatisfactory nature of this situation was recognised by the Law Commission in 1995 when it published its recommendations, including draft legislation (*Law Commission Report No. 231 Mental Incapacity 1995* (HMSO)). Further consultation papers and a White Paper have been published by the Lord Chancellor's Office (1997, 1999).

Basic NHS provisions

The NHS was established on 5 July 1948 under the National Health Service Act 1946. This legislation was re-enacted in the National Health Service Act 1977 which placed the following duties upon the Secretary of State:

Section 1(1)   It is the Secretary of State's duty to continue the promotion in England and Wales of a comprehensive health service designed to secure improvement:
- In the physical and mental health of the people in those countries and
- In the prevention, diagnosis and treatment of illness

And for that purpose to provide and secure the effective provision of services in accordance with this Act.

Section 1(2)   The services so provided shall be free of charge except in so far as the making and recovery of charges is expressly provided for by or under any enactment, whenever passed.

Section 2   Without prejudice to the Secretary of State's powers apart from this section, he has power –
- To provide such services as he considers appropriate for the purpose of discharging any duty imposed on him by this Act; and
- To do any other thing whatsoever which is calculated to facilitate, or is conducive or incidental to, the discharge of such a duty.

This section is subject to section 3 below.

Section 3(1)   It is the Secretary of State's duty to provide throughout England and Wales, to such extent as he considers necessary to meet all reasonable requirements –
- Hospital accommodation;
- Other accommodation for the purpose of any service provided under this Act;
- Medical, dental, nursing and ambulance services;
- Such other facilities for the care of expectant and nursing mothers and young children as he considers are appropriate as part of the health service.

Part II of the Act covers the provision of services by GPs, dental practitioners, pharmacists and others who provide services under a contract for services with the health authorities (which took over responsibilities from the family health service authorities in 1996).

There have been considerable changes in the statutory framework since 1948. The NHS and Community Care Act 1990 led to the establishment of NHS trusts and group fundholding practices. The NHS trusts were to be the principal providers of NHS secondary and community health care. Group fundholding and the internal market (competition between NHS trusts) was abolished in 1999. Under the National Health Service (Primary Care) Act 1997, the Health Act 1999 and the Health and Social Care

Act 2001, primary care trusts (in Wales, local health boards) and care trusts have been established. Since 2002, strategic health authorities have been established, but the primary care trusts are given the spending power for primary, secondary and community services. The NHS Reform and Health Care Professions Act 2002 has facilitated further developments. The White Paper on the NHS incorporated into the Health Act 1999 set out the long-term plans for reorganisation and increased investment in the NHS (DoH 1997). New organisations established since 1999 include the Commission for Health Improvement (CHI) – now amalgamated with the Care Standards Commission in 2003 and now known as the Commission for Health Audit Inspection (CHAI); the National Institute for Clinical Excellence (NICE), the National Patient Safety Agency, the NHS Modernisation Agency, Patient Advocacy and Liaison Services (PALS), Patients' Forums and a Patient Information Advisory Group (Statutory Instrument 2001 No. 2836 Patient Information Advisory Group (Establishment) Regulations 2001) which advises the Secretary of State on the processing of confidential patient information under powers given to the Secretary of State under s.60 Health and Social Care Act 2001. NHS trusts and NHS organisations are required under s.18 Health Act 1999 to comply with a duty of quality that is the statutory basis of the concept of clinical governance. Section 18 states that

> It is the duty of each Health Authority, Primary Care Trust and NHS Trust to put and keep in place arrangements for the purpose of monitoring and improving the quality of health care which it provides to individuals.

Human rights

The European Convention for the Protection of Human Rights and Fundamental Freedoms (1950) provides protection for the fundamental rights and freedoms of all people. The UK is a signatory as are many European countries that are not members of the European Community, for example Norway. The Convention is enforced through the European Commission and the European Court on Human Rights that meets in Strasbourg. However, following the passing of the Human Rights Act 1998 most of the articles are directly enforceable in the UK courts in relation to public authorities or organisations exercising functions of a public nature. As well as placing a duty on public authorities to recognise and implement the articles set out in the convention and in Schedule 1 to the Act, the Act gives a right to individual citizens to bring an action in the courts of the UK if they consider that a public authority has violated their rights. In addition, judges have the power to refer a statute to Parliament if they consider that it is human rights non-compliant. Probably the most significant rights in terms of healthcare are articles 2, 3, 5, 6, 8 and 14. They can be found in Dimond (2001) or at http://www.hmso.legislation.uk.

Law and ethics

Legal principles are ascertainable from legislation or from the decisions in the cases. If a person were to say that X was against the law, then that statement could be verified by finding the appropriate Act of Parliament or statutory instrument or finding the judge's dictum which laid down that particular principle. Ethics, however, relates to a person's upbringing and religion, professional codes of practice or other set of beliefs. A sound legal system should incorporate the ethical beliefs and morality of the majority of the citizens of that country. There are only two situations where the law specifically recognises a conscientious objection: under the Abortion Act 1967 (as amended) and under the Human Fertilisation and Embryology Act 1990, where a person can refuse to participate in a termination or in fertility treatment on grounds of conscientious objection. In the former case, however, this right does not apply if treatment is necessary to save the life or to prevent grave permanent injury to the physical or mental health of a pregnant woman. There may be other situations, however – for example, a Jehovah's Witness nurse who does not wish to care for a woman who is receiving a blood transfusion. In this case, although there is no legal right of refusal, good nursing management would ensure that, if possible, that nurse's ethical views were taken into account in the allocation of patients. If, however, this is managerially impossible, the nurse has no legal right to refuse. The Nursing and Midwifery Council's new Code of Professional Conduct states:

> You must report to a relevant person or authority, at the earliest possible time, any con-
> scientious objection that may be relevant to your professional practice. You must continue to
> provide care to the best of your ability until alternative arrangements are implemented.
> (NMC 2002: clause 2.5)

At the end of this chapter, books are suggested for further reading and discussion on the ethical dimensions of nursing practice.

The four forums of accountability

Where a nurse has caused harm to a patient, the nurse responsible could face legal consequences in several different courts and hearings. If the patient has died, then a report would be made to the coroner, who has the power to decide whether to request a post mortem to be carried out and whether or not an inquest is needed to determine the identity of the deceased and how, when and where that person died. A nurse who is asked to provide a statement to the coroner on an unexpected death should ensure that they have assistance, preferably from a lawyer or from an experienced senior manager in the drafting of this statement, since it is essential to ensure that the statement is clear and comprehensive. A well-written statement may indicate to the coroner that it is not necessary to summon the writer as a witness to the inquest. At any time the coroner can adjourn an inquest and pass the papers to the police and Crown Prosecution Service for criminal proceedings to be investigated.

As well as facing criminal proceedings a nurse could also face civil proceedings where the patient or the relatives of a dead person or child under 18 years are seeking compensation for harm caused by negligence. Disciplinary action by the employer may also follow any incident involving negligent practice by a nurse, and the NMC could also be notified of alleged misconduct and carry out its own investigation leading possibly to a Conduct and Competence Committee hearing. All these courts and hearings are briefly discussed below.

Criminal proceedings

The House of Lords has held that where a health professional acts with such gross negligence that it amounts to a criminal act, then that person can be prosecuted for manslaughter (*R. v. Adomako* House of Lords (1994) 3 All ER 79).

Whilst it is rare for a health professional to be prosecuted in the criminal courts, the possibility of a nurse being summoned to appear as a witness in a colleague's trial is reasonably foreseeable. In such a situation, the actions and records of the nurse would be subjected to scrutiny through cross-examination. The burden is on the prosecution to prove beyond reasonable doubt that the defendant has committed the offence with which they are charged.

Whether an action is a crime or not is dependent upon statute and common law that defines criminal offences. An attempt to commit suicide was a criminal offence prior to the passing of the Suicide Act 1961 but was decriminalised by that Act. However, the Act retained as criminal the offence of aiding and abetting the suicide of another.

Civil proceedings

Any litigant who is seeking to obtain compensation has to establish four elements in the tort (a bundle of civil wrongs) of negligence. They are: that a duty of care was owed to the person who has been harmed; that there has been a breach of this duty of care; and that this breach of duty has caused reasonably foreseeable harm to the claimant. Harm in the form of personal injury or death or loss or damage of property has to be proved. The claimant must prove the existence of these four elements – duty, breach, causation and harm – on a balance of probabilities. Usually the action will be brought against the employer of the negligent person. This is known as the vicarious liability of the employer, and to establish that this applies the claimant will have to show that the person who caused the harm by negligent actions was an employee and was negligent whilst acting in the course of employment. This last phrase has been given an extended meaning by a House of Lords decision (*Lister and Others v. Hesley Hall Ltd*, Times Law Reports, May 10 2001 HL). The employer would probably be vicariously liable even if the employee was failing to obey actual instructions of the employer or working outside her or his competence (*Century Insurance Company Ltd v. Northern Ireland Road Transport Board*, House of Lords (1942) 1 All ER 491).

Disciplinary proceedings

Duty of care

In law there is no duty to volunteer if there is no pre-existing duty. However, the NMC, following the principles set out by the UKCC in its guidelines for professional practice, has retained it as a professional duty for the nurse to accept a 24-hour responsibility. In the new Code of Professional Conduct, the NMC states that:

In an emergency, in or outside the work setting, you have a professional duty to provide care. The care provided would be judged against what could reasonably be expected from someone with your knowledge, skills and abilities when placed in those particular circumstances. (NMC 2002: clause 8.5)

It remains to be seen how the NMC enforces this requirement through its professional conduct machinery. It is unlikely that any trust or other employer would accept liability where a nurse volunteers to take on a duty to help someone when off duty, and so therefore the vicarious liability of the employer would not provide cover for the nurse if she were to cause harm to a person whilst taking on a Good Samaritan role. It is therefore essential that the nurse has professional indemnity cover for such voluntary actions.

Breach of duty

In determining the standard of care that should be followed in healthcare, the courts have used the Bolam Test. This was defined by a judge in a case involving a patient who suffered serious injuries whilst being given electroconvulsive therapy (*Bolam v. Friern Hospital Management Committee* (1957) 1 WLR 582). The judge stated that the standard of care expected is 'the standard of the ordinary skilled man exercising and professing to have that special skill'.

The Bolam Test was applied by the House of Lords in a case where negligence by an obstetrician in delivering a child by forceps was alleged.

When you get a situation which involves the use of some special skill or competence, then the test as to whether there has been negligence or not ... is the standard of the ordinary skilled man exercising and professing to have that special skill. If a surgeon failed to measure up to that in any respect (clinical judgement or otherwise) he had been negligent and should be so adjudged. (*Whitehouse v. Jordan* (1981) 1 All ER 267)

Subsequently the House of Lords in the case of *Bolitho v. City Hospital Hackney Health Authority* (1997) 1 WLR 582 has emphasised the importance of experts giving their opinions to court on the standard of care which should be followed in a specific set of circumstances being reasonable. In this case the House of Lords stated that:

The court had to be satisfied that the exponents of the body of opinion relied on can demonstrate that such opinion has a logical basis. In particular in cases involving, as they often do, the weighing of risks against benefits, the judge, before accepting a body of opinion as being responsible, reasonable or respectable, will need to be satisfied that, in forming their views, the experts had directed their minds to the question of comparative risks and benefits and had reached a defensible conclusion on the matter.

The use of the adjectives 'responsible, reasonable and respectable' [in the Bolam case] all showed that the court had to be satisfied that the exponents of the body of opinion relied upon could demonstrate that such opinion had a logical basis.

It would seldom be right for a judge to reach the conclusion that views held by a competent medical expert were unreasonable.

Increasingly, the Bolam Standards will relate to guidance issued by the National Institute of Clinical Excellence (NICE). Whilst the guidance that this body issues is not legally enforceable, if the guidance is supported by significant research and is shown to be clinically effective then there would be a presumption in favour of its being followed. Each health professional would have to use their own professional discretion in determining the relevance of the guidelines to the particular clinical situation. There is a statutory responsibility on each NHS trust under s.18 Health Act 1999 (see above) to ensure that quality standards are in place and are monitored. In Chapter 5 of this book, clinical practice benchmarking is discussed and it is clear in law that these benchmarks should be regularly reviewed to confirm that they conform to the reasonable standard of care as per the Bolam Test and that individuals use their professional judgement in following them.

Disciplinary proceedings

Each employee has a contract of employment that sets out express terms to be observed by both employer and employee. In addition, terms are implied by the courts that are considered intrinsic to a contract of employment. These require the employee to act with reasonable care and skill and to obey reasonable instructions, and the employer to take reasonable care of the health and safety of the employee. If the employee should fail to observe these implied terms, then the employer can take disciplinary action against the employee, the final sanction being dismissal.

The employee (if they satisfy the necessary legal requirements) can apply to an employment tribunal to challenge a dismissal. If the employee is injured as a result of failures by the employer to fulfil its contractual duty, then the employee can sue for compensation in the civil courts for breach of the implied term in the contract of employment, or if the employee fears that injury is likely and the employer fails to take reasonable action to prevent injury, then the employee could claim that they have been subject to constructive dismissal because the employer is in fundamental breach of the contract of employment.

Reasonable instructions

As stated above, it is an implied term in the contract of employment that an employee must obey the reasonable instructions of the employer. The job description is seen not as a contractual term (which would mean that it could be changed only by agreement between the parties) but as within the control of the employer to alter as necessary. If an advanced practitioner received what they felt to be unreasonable instructions by the employer, what is the legal situation? For example, they may be asked to undertake activities for which they consider that they have not had the training and which are, therefore, outside their competence. The advanced practitioner would have to show the employer why the instructions were unreasonable and be constructive regarding the necessary action to ensure their competence. There would be advantages in their putting this in writing.

Whistle-blowing

Where an advanced practitioner is concerned that unacceptable or dangerous practices are taking place in the trust, that nurse should ensure that a report is made to the appropriate manager. If there is a failure to take action, then the advanced practitioner should use the procedure set up by their employer under the Public Interest Disclosure Act 1998 to ensure that these concerns are raised at the highest level within the organisation and that action is taken to remedy them (HSC 1999/198 Public Interest Disclosure Act 1998). The Kennedy report on paediatric heart surgery at Bristol Royal Infirmary made some radical recommendations on developing an honest, open culture within the NHS where patients and professionals worked in partnership.

Professional proceedings

Nursing and Midwifery Council

In April 2002 the Nursing and Midwifery Council (NMC) took over its responsibilities as a registration body, having operated in shadow format alongside the UKCC for almost a year. During that time it had agreed with the UKCC a revised code of professional conduct that came into force in June 2002. The new Code replaces the earlier Code of Professional Conduct, the *Guidelines for Professional Practice* and the *Scope of Professional Practice*. It has been reviewed by Dimond (2002a), who has suggested possible improvements. The NMC itself welcomes, from both registered practitioners and the public, any feedback on the Code so that amendments can be made.

Professional conduct proceedings

Four practice committees have been set up under the NMC for the determination of fitness to practise and professional misconduct. They are the Preliminary Proceedings (Investigating) Committee, the Professional Conduct and Competence Committee, the Health Committee and the Midwifery Committee. Screeners are appointed to carry out the initial investigation of any allegation against a registered practitioner. The basic procedures for these committees are laid down by statutory instrument and, at this early stage in the life of the NMC, it is uncertain how the Council will exercise its control over registered practitioners in comparison with its predecessor the UKCC. The ultimate sanction over the registered practitioner is to be struck off the Register, but there are many other powers of the NMC, including issuing a caution and suspension from the Register.

Under the NHS Reform and Health Care Professions Act 2002, a Council for the Regulation of Health Care Professionals is to be established which will have the functions of: promoting the interests of patients and other members of the public in relation to the performance of their functions by the various professional registration bodies; promoting best practice in the performance of those functions; formulating principles relating to good professional self-regulation and encouraging regulatory bodies to conform to them; and promoting cooperation between regulatory bodies and between them, or any of them, and other bodies performing corresponding functions. The new Council is likely to increase the uniformity between the different professional regulation bodies.

Scope of professional practice

Unless an Act of Parliament or other statutory provision requires an activity to be undertaken by a specific health professional, then, provided the necessary training, experience and knowledge are acquired so that the activity could be undertaken competently, any registered health professional could undertake that activity. One of the very few statutes that require particular activities to be performed only by a practitioner of a specified registered profession is the Mental Health Act 1983. The Abortion Act 1967 requires an approved termination to be carried out by a registered medical practitioner, but the House of Lords interpreted this as meaning that the doctor responsible for the termination when prostaglandins were being administered could supervise its being carried out by a nurse (*Royal College of Nursing of the UK v. Department of Health and Social Security* (1981) AC 800: 1981 1 All ER 545). As Lord Diplock said in the House of Lords:

> [The] doctor need not do everything with his own hands; the subsection's requirements were satisfied when the treatment was one prescribed by a registered medical practitioner carried out in accordance with his directions and of which he remained in charge throughout.

The Medicines Act 1968 also specifies which named professions can undertake activities under the Act, but community nurse prescribing was permitted under legislation – the Medicinal Products: Prescription by Nurses etc. Act 1992. A statutory instrument was published in 2000 specifying the minimum requirements for a patient group direction (originally known as group protocol). Subsequently, s.63 Health and Social Care Act 2001 (Prescription Only Medicines (Human Use) Amendment Order 2000 SI 2000 No. 1917) has extended the provisions of s.58 Medicines Act 1968 to enable other registered health practitioners to have prescribing powers. Regulations were enacted in 2002 specifying the conditions under which these practitioners can prescribe and what they can prescribe (Statutory Instrument 2002 No. 549 Prescription Only Medicines (Human Use) Amendment Order 2000). Nurse prescribing is considered in Chapter 14 of this book.

Where there is no specific statutory requirement that only specified registered practitioners can carry out an activity, then provided health professionals have the necessary training, experience, knowledge and competence, they can in law undertake that activity even though the activity is usually associated with another professional. This gives enormous flexibility to working practices, but could also lead to overlaps and gaps in professional practice. For example the Audit Commission report on anaesthetics pointed out that many different health professionals could undertake the same activities in the operating theatre and recovery room and it was important to clarify responsibilities and standards (Audit Commission 1997). It is a legal principle that where another professional group undertakes activities formerly undertaken by a different profession, a lower standard is not acceptable: the same reasonable standard of care must be provided.

Whilst the *Scope of Professional Practice* issued by the UKCC has now been replaced by the new Code of Professional Conduct, the guidelines for developing the scope laid down by the Council are still relevant and of value to the nurse practitioner. They are shown in Table 15.1.

Table 15.1   Principles for adjusting the *Scope of Professional Practice*

The registered nurse, midwife or health visitor:
(1)   Must be satisfied that each aspect of practice is directed to meeting the needs and serving the interests of the patient or client
(2)   Must endeavour always to achieve, maintain and develop knowledge, skill and competence to respond to those needs and interests
(3)   Must honestly acknowledge any limits of personal knowledge and skill and take steps to remedy any relevant deficits in order effectively and appropriately to meet the needs of patients and clients
(4)   Must ensure that any enlargement or adjustment of the scope of personal professional practice must be achieved without compromising or fragmenting existing aspects of professional practice and care and that requirements of the Council's Code of Professional Conduct are satisfied throughout the whole area of practice
(5)   Must recognise and honour the direct or indirect personal accountability borne for all aspects of professional practice
(6)   Must, in serving the interests of patients and clients and the wider interests of society, avoid any inappropriate delegation to others which compromises those interests

Nurse consultants

There is no statutory provision for the establishment of nurse consultants, so there is no legal limit or legal specification for their role (other than that which applies to all health professionals, for example the Medicines Act 1968, the Mental Health Act 1983 – see above). The NHS Plan envisaged that 1000 nurse consultants would be appointed. The key features of the nurse consultant were set out in *Making a Difference* (DoH 1999a), and are:

- Expert practice
- Professional leadership and consultancy
- Education and development
- Practice and service development linked to research and evaluation.

It is envisaged that at least half of the nurse consultant's time will be spent on clinical work with career opportunities. NHS trusts are required to agree the posts with regional offices of the DoH.

It is the personal and professional responsibility of nurse consultants to ensure that they work within the scope of their professional practice and to refuse to undertake those activities that are outside their competence. The law does not accept any principle of team liability. Whilst collaboration and multidisciplinary working are essential in healthcare, ultimately each member of the team is personally accountable for their own actions. It is important to be aware of the fact that the law does not recognise a lowering of standards when activities are undertaken by nurses rather than doctors. The patient is entitled to the reasonable standard of care as per the Bolam Test (see earlier), whichever professional undertakes the work.

Clinical nurse specialists and specialist nurses

Nurses who take on these specialists' responsibilities need to clarify their responsibilities and ensure that they are acting within the boundaries of their competence. Protocols may often be drawn up and agreed by the multidisciplinary team and senior management on the role to be performed by the specialist. The nurse is entitled to insist on receiving the necessary training and/or supervised practice before taking on specialist responsibilities. It is also essential that they agree with other health professional colleagues such as doctors, physiotherapists, and others, how their work interacts to ensure that there are no gaps or duplications in patient care. Where the specialist is entitled to receive direct referrals of patients then it is essential that there is clear identification of those conditions that would be deemed to be outside the specialist's jurisdiction.

NHS Direct

NHS Direct was one of the first of the innovations introduced by the Labour government for the NHS and initially operated on a restricted basis. The White Paper on the NHS proposed the establishment of NHS Direct. The government's aim was that by the end of the year 2000 the whole country would be covered by a 24-hour telephone advice line staffed by nurses (DoH 1997). A director was appointed for NHS Direct in Wales that became operational in January 2000.

The service aims to provide both clinical advice to support self-care and appropriate self-referral to NHS services as well as access to more general advice and information. NHS Direct is now linking up with out-of-hours services to provide a triage assessment for out-of-hours visits by doctors.

Walk-in clinics

Direct access clinics run by nurses, to which any person can go for assistance and advice on healthcare, were set up in 1999. They aim, in the words of the press release,

> to offer quick access to a range of NHS services including free consultations, minor treatments, health information and advice on self-treatment. They are based in convenient locations that allow the public easy access and have opening hours tailored to suit modern lifestyles, including early mornings, late evenings, and weekends. The centres will have close links with local GPs ensuring continuity of care for their patients. (DoH 1999b)

The advantages to the public are apparent: fast service, no wait, close to work, easy access, immediate advice, speedy prescriptions. Many of the clinics are planned to be linked with GP surgeries through information technology.

In February 2000, the classification of nurses who could have powers to prescribe in the community was extended by Statutory Instrument 2000 No. 121 The National Health Service (Pharmaceutical Services) Amendment Regulations 2000 to include nurses employed by a doctor whose name is included in a medical list (i.e. practice nurses) and those assisting in the capacity of a nurse, in the provision of services in a 'walk-in centre' which in this regulation means a centre at which information and treatment for minor conditions is provided to the public under arrangements made by or on behalf of the Secretary of State.

Delegation and supervision

Inevitably, as the nurse practitioner takes on an expanded role, then an increased number of activities must be delegated to other healthcare support workers. Legal liability can result if these activities are delegated inappropriately or if there is inadequate supervision. The delegating nurse must ensure themself of the competence of the person who is carrying out activities that they would usually have performed and provide the level of supervision to ensure that the patient is reasonably safe. The person undertaking the delegated task must ensure that the reasonable standard of care is followed (i.e. the Bolam test – see above).

If the advanced practitioner has delegated appropriately and provided the correct level of supervision, then they would not be liable if the health support worker was negligent and caused harm in carrying out their duties. In this context the word 'supervision' is used in a management sense, i.e. it is the responsibility of management to ensure that activities are appropriately delegated and that there is the correct level of supervision. In Chapter 6 of this book, which considers supervision and leadership, the word 'supervision' is used in the sense of mentorship and support. The UKCC supported the use of clinical supervision as reflective practice. Clearly the legal implications of management supervision are very different from the legal issues that arise from the role of a supervisor. Further discussion of this issue is considered in Dimond (2001).

Patient rights

Right to services

Patients do not have an absolute right to access services. As is seen above, the statutory duty placed upon the Secretary of State is to provide a reasonable service. These duties have been considered by the courts in a number of different cases and the general consensus is that the statute does not give an absolute right to obtain services, and that, provided there is no obvious evidence of irrational or unreasonable setting of priorities, then the courts will not be involved in the determination of the allocation of resources (*R. v. Secretary of State for Social Services ex parte Hincks and others*, 29 June 1979 (1979) 123 Solicitors Journal 436).

Right to consent

A mentally competent adult has a right to give or refuse consent to any treatment, even if it is life-saving. A young person of 16 or 17 has a statutory right to give consent under s.8 Family Law Reform Act 1969, but this does not include the right to refuse life-saving treatment (*Re. W (minor) (medical treatment)* (1992) 4 All ER 627). Children under 16 have a right, recognised at common law, to give consent if they are deemed Gillick competent. This principle was established by the House of Lords in *Gillick v. West Norfolk and Wisbech AHA and the DHSS* (1985) 3 All ER 402. Decisions can be made in the best interests of the mentally incapacitated adult under powers recognised by the House of Lords (*Re. F. (mental patient: sterilisation)* (1990) 2 AC 1). In Scotland there is statutory provision to cover decision-making on behalf of the mentally incapacitated adult, but in England, Wales and Northern Ireland legislation must await the outcome of the consultation process on the Mental Health Bill 2002. Further details on this area can be found in Dimond (2002b).

Right to confidentiality

Every patient is entitled to have their confidentiality respected and it is the professional duty of the health professional to ensure that this is implemented. A practitioner could face criminal, civil, disciplinary and professional conduct proceedings if confidentiality is not respected. The Data Protection Act 1998 applies to both manually held and computerised records and lays down the principles for the keeping of patient-identifiable information. There are, in law, certain exceptions recognised to the duty of confidentiality, including disclosure in the public interest. This exception is also recognised in the Code of Professional Conduct of the NMC. The practitioner is personally responsible for ensuring that any disclosure is justified and for recording the fact of the disclosure and its reasons. Further details on this area can be found in Dimond (2002c).

Right of access to records

Under statutory regulations drawn up under the Data Protection Act 1998, every person is entitled to access their personal health records. The right is not, however, absolute and access can be withheld if serious harm would be caused to the physical or mental health or condition of the applicant or another person, or if a third person (not being the health professional caring for the patient) would be identified by the disclosure and has asked not to be identified.

Right to complain

A system for handling complaints in hospitals and in the community has been in existence in the NHS since 1996 following the Wilson Report (DoH 1994). The present system involves a three-stage process: local resolution, an independent review panel and appeal to the Health Service Commissioner. Several years ago research was commissioned by the Department of Health on the effectiveness of the current complaints system. In the light of the results of that research, the Department of Health published a document suggesting a number of ways to improve the current procedure (DoH 2001a). It also issued a consultation document on which feedback was invited. It is likely to lead to significant changes to the present complaints system (DoH 2001b).

Record-keeping

Clear, comprehensive record-keeping is part of the professional responsibilities of the nurse practitioner. It therefore follows that one of the duties of the advanced nurse practitioner would be to ensure that patient records comply with the standards set by the NMC and that action is taken to ensure that there is regular audit of standards of documentation. Records relating to the advanced practice itself, role definition and specification, and clinical supervision records would also need to be kept.

Conclusion

Individual practitioners are personally and professionally accountable for their practice. If they are working at advanced levels they must personally ensure that they have the competence to perform those activities at the reasonable standard of those originally entrusted with those duties. They are also personally responsible for ensuring that their competence is maintained and they obtain the necessary supervised practice and study leave.

Where it is necessary to delegate activities, then such delegation and the level of supervision provided must accord with reasonable standards of care. The developments in advanced nursing practice present formidable challenges for NMC practitioners. The problems that arise are considerable, but so also are the opportunities.

References

Audit Commission (1997) *Anaesthesia Under Examination: The Efficiency and Effectiveness of Anaesthesia and Pain Relief Services in England and Wales.* London: Audit Commission.

Dimond, B. (2001) *Legal Aspects of Nursing*, 3rd edn. Harlow: Pearson Education.

Dimond, B. (2002a) The new code of professional conduct. *British Journal of Midwifery*, 10 (7): 456–9.

Dimond, B. (2002b) *The Legal Aspects of Consent.* Dinton: Quay Publications.

Dimond, B. (2002c) *The Legal Aspects of Confidentiality.* Dinton: Quay Publications.

DoH (1994) *Being Heard. The Report of the Review Committee on NHS Complaints Procedures,* chaired by Professor Alan Wilson, May 1994.

DoH (1997) *The New NHS: Modern, Dependable.* London: DoH.

DoH (1999a) *Making a Difference: Strengthening the Nursing, Midwifery and Health Visiting Contribution to Health and Healthcare.* London, DOH.

DoH (1999b) Press release. *Frank Dobson Announces More NHS Walk-in Clinics.* London: DoH.
DoH (2001a) *The NHS Complaints Procedure: National Evaluation.* Leeds: DoH.
DoH (2001b) *Reforming the NHS Complaints Procedure: A Listening Document.* Leeds: DoH.
Lord Chancellor's Office (1997) *Who Decides?* London: The Stationery Office.
Lord Chancellor's Office (1999) *Making Decisions.* London: The Stationery Office.
NMC (2002) *Code of Professional Conduct.* London: NMC.

Further reading

Brazier, M. (1992) *Medicine, Patients and the Law.* London: Penguin.
Brazier, M. & Murphy, J. (eds) (1999) *The Law of Torts,* 10th edn. London: Butterworth.
Card, R. (1998) *Card, Cross and Jones' Criminal Law,* 14th edn. London: Butterworth.
Dimond, B.C. (1999) *Patients' Rights, Responsibilities and the Nurse,* 2nd edn. Dinton: Quay Publications.
Dimond, B.C. (2002) *Legal Aspects of Midwifery,* 2nd edn. Oxford: Books for Midwives Press.
Dimond, B.C. (1997) *Legal Aspects of Care in the Community.* Basingstoke: Macmillan.
Dimond, B.C. (1998) *Legal Aspects of Complementary Therapy Practice.* Edinburgh: Churchill Livingstone.
Dimond, B.C. (2002) *Legal Aspects of Pain Management.* Dinton: Quay Publications.
Harris, P. (1997) *An Introduction to Law,* 5th edn. London: Butterworth.
Heywood Jones, I. (ed.) (1999) *The UKCC Code of Conduct: A Critical Guide.* London: Nursing Times Books.
Hunt, G. & Wainwright, P. (eds) (1994) *Expanding the Role of the Nurse.* Oxford: Blackwell Science.
Hurwitz, B. (1998) *Clinical Guidelines and the Law.* Oxford: Radcliffe Medical Press.
Kennedy, I. & Grubb, A. (2000) *Medical Law and Ethics,* 3rd edn. London: Butterworth.
Kloss, D. (2000) *Occupational Health Law,* 3rd edn. Oxford: Blackwell Science.
Mandelstam, M. (1998) *An A–Z of Community Care Law.* London: Jessica Kingsley.
Markesinis, B.S. & Deakin, S.F. (1999) *Tort Law,* 4th edn. Oxford: Clarendon Press.
Mason, J.K. & McCall-Smith, A. (1999) *Law and Medical Ethics,* 5th edn. London: Butterworth.
McHale, J., Fox, M., with Murphy, J. (1997) *Health Care Law.* London: Sweet & Maxwell.
McHale, J., Tingle J. & Peysner, J. (1998) *Law and Nursing.* Oxford: Butterworth-Heinemann.
Montgomery, J. (1997) *Health Care Law.* Oxford: Oxford University Press.
National Association of Theatre Nurses (1993) *The Role of the Nurse as First Assistant in the Operating Department.* Harrogate: NATN.
Pitt, G. (2000) *Employment Law,* 4th edn. London: Sweet & Maxwell.
Rowson, R. (1990) *Introduction to Ethics for Nurses.* London: Scutari Press.
Rumbold, G. (1999) *Ethics in Nursing Practice,* 2nd edn. Edinburgh: Baillière Tindall/RCN.
Selwyn, N. (2000) *Selwyn's Law of Employment,* 11th edn, London: Butterworth.
Sims, S. (2000) *Practical Approach to Civil Procedure,* 4th edn. London: Blackstone Press.
Skegg, P.D.G. (1998) *Law, Ethics and Medicine,* 2nd edn. Oxford: Oxford University Press.
Tschudin, V. & Marks-Maran, D. (1993) *Ethics: A Primer for Nurses.* London: Baillière-Tindall.
Vincent, C. (ed.) (1995) *Clinical Risk Management.* London: BMJ Publications.
Wilkinson, R. & Caulfield, H. (2000) *The Human Rights Act: A Practical Guide for Nurses.* London: Whurr.

Chapter 16

The Political Context of Advanced Nursing Practice

George Castledine

Introduction

The global agenda for nursing provided by the World Health Organisation (WHO) is intended to bring about improvements in health through the development of roles that increase access to healthcare, particularly for vulnerable and socially excluded populations (WHO 2000). In setting this agenda, WHO has left each country free to develop approaches that meet the needs of their populations. Inevitably, debating and deciding appropriate courses of action brings healthcare into the political arena through which the state determines the nature and objectives of service and the ways in which professionals will function to deliver these. Thus politics in this context is about the democratic exercise of power and the formation of policy from debate. Advanced practice represents one strategy for achieving the WHO agenda within the UK. It provides opportunities for the creative application of nursing expertise in new professional territories and in ways that enhance the health of both individuals and populations. Advanced practitioners are agents of change, the leaders in their fields of practice: a factor that requires them to become astute in their understanding and exercise of influence and power to motivate others to bring about change.

Despite the emergence of feminism and the increase in higher education for nurses, nursing has not emerged as a political force in the UK. Sociologists still define nursing as a 'semi-profession' and the public are still not sure where nursing stands in relation to medicine. Perhaps because of the image of nursing as a subordinate and largely silent profession, fewer young people of either sex are opting for it as a career and the result is a potentially calamitous national shortage of nurses. The government in the UK has taken over the professional voice of nursing and because of its national health strategy has decided what the direction for nurses will be. This aggressive move may help shake nursing out of its doldrums and encourage new political nursing leaders to emerge, especially among those working in advanced nursing practice. On the other hand, it may reinforce the relatively accepted powerless state of nursing as a low-status group in healthcare. If nursing is to take on a more visionary and activist role, advanced nurse practitioners will need the backing of nursing's professional orga-nisations or a group that specially supports their political endeavours. This chapter begins by examining and tracing the political context in which advanced practice has developed, drawing on historical and contemporary sources. It goes on to address ways in which the advanced practitioner can become more active in the political arena at local, regional and national levels. The chapter draws to a close by considering some of the key political issues that will need to be addressed in the near future.

The political context in which advanced nursing practice has developed

Politics and social policy play major roles in shaping the current and emerging state of healthcare in the UK. It is the state's responsibility to provide a health and social care service which is accessible, provides a reasonable quality of care and treatment, and is fair to all.

In medieval England, it was not considered to be the responsibility of the state to look after the poor and sick. It was the Church that took on this role and which encouraged the more wealthy to set a good example by contributing large sums of money to cover the costs. Monasteries also helped to take care of the sick and poor, and sometimes an almoner was appointed to distribute alms of food or money. It was the religious almoners who probably formed the first health and social services to people in the community. In the peaceful and fairly prosperous conditions of the twelfth and thirteenth centuries, kings and bishops, wealthy merchants and municipal guilds followed the teaching of the Church and founded charitable institutions or bequeathed land to endow charitable foundations. Many of these foundations were hospitals (Daltrop 1978). Medieval hospitals were places of general hospitality; their services were for the old and needy and for travellers too poor to afford an inn, as well as for the sick.

Two of the most famous of London's present-day hospitals for the sick were founded by religious communities during the twelfth century: St Bartholomew's and St Thomas'. Hospitals began to spring up across Europe along the busy pilgrim routes, but not all were intended for hospitality for pilgrims. There were almshouses for the aged and infirm, orphanages, lying-in hospitals for women and leper hospitals. Eventually, separate establishments were developed for the mentally sick, insane or mentally defective.

Throughout the centuries, charitable individuals, societies and associations were formed to help the sick and poor. The great voluntary hospital movement in Britain began in the eighteenth century, and money to support such institutions was raised mainly by voluntary donations and subscriptions. With the advent of the Industrial Revolution, life for many people in Britain changed dramatically. Technology and business led the way as thousands of people flocked into London, Birmingham, Liverpool and Manchester from the surrounding countryside to work in the factories. But with this mass migration of people and the development of crowded, smoky, filthy working conditions, came new health problems. Many employers in those days believed that the working classes must be taught thrift, industry, temperance and family responsibility. Very few provided many welfare and health facilities for their workers, preferring to encourage those who could, to save in a friendly society or resort to charity in an emergency. The range of Victorian charities in Britain was immense and formed a strong tradition, which thrives to this day.

Forty specialist voluntary hospitals were founded in London between 1820 and 1860, including eye, ear, heart and children's hospitals. In Liverpool a local merchant named William Rathbone founded the District Nursing Association. There is no doubt that the great age of medical specialisation had begun and was established in the nineteenth century through the foundation of the specialist hospital. Charity became fashionable and received state approval through royal patronage and local members of Parliament.

Unfortunately, despite the increase in the wealth of the country, and some individuals in particular, the poor were getting poorer and the number of sick people was increasing. This led two men, Charles Booth and Seebohm Rowntree, to study the seriousness of the situation and produce social survey reports that had a great impact upon the politicians and policy-makers of the time. Very soon a Royal Commission was set up to examine the operation of the Poor Law system. Between 1906 and 1914 a national welfare state came into being as the Liberal government passed legislation providing for old age pensions, labour exchanges, unemployment and sickness insurance, school health services and meals for schoolchildren, and remand homes and juvenile courts for children in trouble. By 1914, the main responsibility for the welfare of the underprivileged had shifted from private charity to the state.

More emphasis on state intervention for the poor and sick followed, and the National Health Service was introduced in 1948. It was thought that with the introduction of the new welfare state, charities would disappear. This certainly was the case in some European countries such as Scandinavia, but in Britain the traditions continued to the present day. There was always the doubt about whether the welfare state's provisions were working as well as people expected, and by the 1950s and 1960s new charities, such as the Spastics Society in 1952, Shelter in 1966 and St Christopher's Hospice for palliative care in London in 1967, were being developed to meet perceived gaps in state provision.

The role of charities today

With government becoming more complex and centralised there is a danger that local needs are ignored and minority groups in health and welfare become remote and sidelined. It is to their credit, therefore, that charities in the UK persevere and take on areas and services that the state is never likely to take over, providing not only an alternative to mainstream healthcare but, in some instances, the only service for those with special health and social needs. They represent the values of a society and are essential for maintaining standards of compassion and protection of the weak and disadvantaged. There is a very special role for the voluntary worker in the welfare of the country, and many healthcare organisations encourage their participation as it often helps in making scarce resources go further, allowing professional staff to direct their time to areas of greatest need. Working closely with charities is, therefore, a key element of government policy, and advanced practitioners should be aware of the need to do likewise, carefully weighing up where and how volunteers can best be used, supported or developed. Volunteers may well have experienced first-hand the problems with which patients are trying to come to terms. Sharing such experiences can provide patients with a source of help that is outside professional expertise. Such sharing may also have a therapeutic value, enabling the volunteer to gain in self-esteem by helping others.

Nursing's political realisation

Politics is about the exercise of power and authority. Nurses often shy away from politics because they feel it is too far removed from them and not specific enough to affairs that affect them directly. Politics is, however, also about belonging to, or taking an interest in things that matter to us, the groups and organisations we belong to, and the status and influence they exert on society.

The history of the modern nursing movement is generally accredited to Florence Nightingale because she opened the nurse-training programme at St Thomas' Hospital in England in 1860. Before this time there was very little formal training of nurses anywhere in the world. Where it did exist it was often closely linked to religious orders, and was carried out at the bedside. Nursing, long considered women's work, shared with the overall women's movement the many negative, devalued perceptions of the worth of its role (Vance *et al.* 1985; Reverby 1987). As a result of such a perception, nursing suffers from 'nursism' (Lewenson 2002), which has been defined as a form of sexism that specifically maligns the caring role in society. The public's perception of the nurse has changed little over the years and is still seen as an assistant to the doctor or as a job done by those who have a natural flair for caring. The notion that 'nurses are born, not made' persists in the twenty-first century and has provided a rationale for hiring less-educated workers to perform professional nursing roles. This rationale is evident in current UK health policy that directs more educated nurses towards medicalised roles and delegates more basic care such as washing or feeding patients, to healthcare assistants. Elsewhere, for example in the USA, hospitals routinely reduce costs by firing nurses with experience and advanced degrees and cross-train uneducated healthcare workers to do jobs once done by registered nurses. This acceptance of less-qualified nurses reflects the decreased value society continues to place on professional nursing care.

Lewenson (2002) argues that nursing was one of the first professions that women sought to control and organise. This was particularly so in North America and rose out of the political efforts of women during what is known as the Woman Movement of the mid-nineteenth and early twentieth centuries. Nightingale believed that nurses should control their own profession. She used a variety of strategies to convey her views, and among the most effective was her passion for writing letters to influential people. It was this 'political' pressure that got her ideas about sanitation, education and the separation of nursing and medicine, accepted around the world. An editorial comment published in the *American Journal of Nursing* (1908) acknowledged that her 'brilliant essence lay in her taking from men's hands a power which did not logically or rightly belong to them, but which they had usurped, and seizing it firmly as her own, from whence she passed it on to her pupils and disciples'. Nightingale's ideas on separating nursing and medicine were instrumental in many countries in reforming the deplorable conditions found in hospitals. It seems ironic that, in the UK, nurses are now being encouraged to integrate more closely with medicine and give up their basic caring role in order to help the health service get through its medical staffing crises and meet its medical objectives. Nursing in the UK is, therefore, in danger of becoming too specialised along medical guidelines, and losing its general holistic caring function.

The political role of individuals and professional organisations

Various professional nursing organisations came into existence around the late 1880s and early 1900s. It was no coincidence that many of these groups were heavily influenced by some of the strong characters and personalities in nursing at the time. Ethel Bedford Fenwick (1857–1947) was matron of St Bartholomew's Hospital from 1881 to 1897. She strongly disapproved of people being nursed by the untrained, and devoted her life's work to the professional status of nursing. She formed the British Nurses' Association, which was the first organisation of professional nurses. The first meeting took place in her house in 1887. Membership was not limited to trained nurses, but included medical men, some of whom were even honorary officers. The Association grew rapidly and after one year had some 1000 members. Bedford Fenwick did not get on with Nightingale and there was often disagreement between them. In 1892, however, a Royal Charter was issued and the organisation became known as the Royal British Nurses' Association.

Once the Royal British Nurses' Association had shown the advantages of a nurses' organisation, similar societies sprung up both in Britain and in the rest of the world. The history and development of nurses' associations has not always been consistent or easy to trace. In North America, for instance, each training school formed an alumnae association, with national organisations emerging later. In Britain, at the time, alumnae associations came a close second in professional nursing organisation development and were known as hospital leagues or fellowships. Their political influence was much less than that of the national associations and they existed more so that nurses might keep in touch with each other and the hospital in which they had trained.

Sarah Swift (born in 1854, and a former matron of several hospitals, including Guy's Hospital, London) was the motivator behind the formation of the College of Nursing in 1916. This became the Royal College of Nursing in 1939. She saw nursing issues differently from both Nightingale and Bedford Fenwick and, along with Rachael Annie Cox-Davies, the matron of the Royal Free Hospital who launched the Association of Hospital Matrons in 1919, established the College of Nursing 'to provide a uniform standard of training ... to improve the quality of the nursing service, and the conditions under which nurses work, to assist in the securing of State Registration of Nurses, and to further in every possible way the advancement of the profession through legislation, post-graduate study, theoretical and practical scholarships and specialised training' (Bowman 1967). Although launched during the First World War, the value of the College was soon apparent and within a few years its membership reached the thousands (Bowman 1967).

Today the Royal College of Nursing (RCN) is the largest professional body for nurses in the UK. It has survived because it has adapted to the needs of its members. Like other national associations in other countries, it is of paramount importance for nursing. During the early years of specialisation it was the RCN which first responded to the needs of nurses undertaking new roles. For example, the case for an advanced clinical role for the nurse in the UK was originally put forward by the RCN and discussed at a special seminar held at Leeds Castle in Kent (RCN 1975). Since that time the RCN policy has been to encourage and support the development of new roles. There has been a dramatic increase in the number of specialist entities belonging to the RCN, many of these specialist groups following traditional medical specialities. However, some specialist nursing groups, such as the Association of Theatre Nurses and the Infection Control Nurses' Association, have remained outside the College's network. There is no doubt that specialist interest groups and organisations can play a significant part in putting political pressure on both internal and external nursing policy-makers. What seems key in this is the emergence of new visionary nurse leaders with a specific interest in the future role of advanced nurse practitioners.

The politics of regulation

The purpose of any governmental regulation of professional practice, including nursing, is the protection of the public. Usually, when considering whether a profession or occupation should be regulated, certain criteria are used such as: the potential risk of harm to the consumer, whether or not specialised education is required, the complexity of skills and knowledge, and the level of autonomy required of the provider (Hutcherson 2002). Nursing shared common characteristics for professionalisation with other Victorian and Edwardian groups, including medicine, midwifery, dentistry, teaching and accountancy. The process of state registration of nurses, which was the cornerstone of regulation, was very much a 'protracted campaign, sectional, bitter and divisive' (Abel-Smith 1960; Maggs 1983). There were those leading nurses such as Bedford Fenwick, who were for it, and those such as Nightingale, who were against it. Some of those who argued against registration did so on the basis that it would narrow the field of recruitment to nursing, the fee would be prohibitive, the educational standard of a nurse did not need to be raised too high, and, as Sydney Holland was quoted as saying, 'we want to stop nurses thinking themselves anything more than they are, namely the faithful carriers out of the doctor's orders' (Abel-Smith 1960). Despite all this, state registration was introduced in 1919 by the government of the day.

Gaining legal recognition for the establishment of a register of qualified nurses, plus deciding on appropriate initial education and restricting practice to those whose competence is recognised through registration, lies at the heart of what is known as professional self-regulation (PSR). Over the years, there have been some changes to this process for nurses. The Nurses Act 1919 gave statutory recognition to those nurses who met certain requirements for registration as a nurse. At first the General Register was open only to women nurses, and therefore there were supplementary registers for men, for those who had trained in the nursing of the mentally sick, of the mentally subnormal, the nursing of sick children and of fevers. Over time, these branches of nursing became more highly specialised and the theoretical context more complex, thus there was pressure for change. This led to the supplementary part of the Register for male nurses being merged with the General Register. In 1979 the Nurses, Midwives and Health Visitors Act heralded far-reaching changes in the regulation of nurses. The new Act brought together nine bodies previously responsible, in whole or in part, for separate regulation of midwifery, health visiting and nursing within the UK.

The United Kingdom Central Council for Nursing, Midwifery and Health Visiting (UKCC) and four national boards established by the new Act, created by far the largest regulatory body for any healthcare profession. It also resulted in the largest register of its kind for nurses, midwives and health visitors in the world. In the early days, the Council or ruling body of the UKCC was elected through the national boards, but towards the end of its reign, the last two councils were democratically elected from the nurses themselves in the four countries of England, Wales, Scotland and Northern Ireland.

During the 1990s, regulatory bodies such as the UKCC and the General Medical Council faced new and more stringent political questioning. This included public questions over rulings made on removing doctors and nurses from, and restoring them to, the relevant registers. Several high-profile cases involving doctors and nurses resulted in doubts over the value of self-regulation and the need for more public involvement (Davies & Beach 2000). By 2002, therefore, the Labour government had reviewed the regulation of the healthcare professions and decided that a new regulatory board would be introduced. This body was called the Nursing and Midwifery Council (NMC) and represented a dramatic reduction in democratically elected members of the professions and an increase in members of the public.

The regulation of advanced practice

Following the introduction of the advanced role, nurses and members of other professions expressed concerns that some of those professing to be working in advanced practice were or might be practising beyond their ability and scope. There was also some evidence that, in the absence of clear descriptors or competences for the role, some nurses were using the term 'advanced practitioner' as a job title rather than a level of practice. The absence of a uniform national standard for advanced practice nurses resulted in confusion for the public, managers and other healthcare providers about the role and authority of such practitioners. Therefore it was no surprise when the UKCC set up a working group not only to identify what were the criteria and competences of advanced practice, but also to work towards formally recognising and regulating this level of practice.

The group was set up in the late 1990s and used the term 'higher-level practice' (HLP) to denote the level of practice that was being examined, and to avoid any initial confusion with the term 'advanced practice'. When the final report (UKCC 2002) was published it laid out a standard and criteria for higher-level practice that had been piloted and tested by an external research team (City & Guilds Affinity). The result was very positive and demonstrated not only a national standard but also a useful framework for identifying and recognising those nurses working at an advanced level.

The UKCC's work also contributed to the consultant nurse (midwife/health visitor) initiatives in the UK and is being used by employers to structure job descriptions, inform educationalists for future courses and risk managers of the legal and professional implications of expanding nurses' roles. It also recommended that there should be national regulation of advanced practice. However, to date no system has been established to regulate advanced practice

Nurses, nursing and the politics of healthcare

There is no doubt that the role and position of nurses and nursing in the development of healthcare in the UK today has never been more challenging. The NHS is a major weapon in any political party, and the current Labour government is not only committed to modernising the health service, but is also determined that it will succeed with its plans. Several key strategies are central to the government's reforms for the NHS, and it is important that specialist nurses and advanced practitioners are aware of them.

Spending in the old NHS was something of an annual lottery; now there are tighter spending plans and targets which are regularly reviewed. Management of the old NHS was often dictated by the fancies and whims of individuals; now there is the introduction of general managers and boards of directors in an effort to promote sound modern-day management principles. Before, there were no national standards for medical care and treatment; now, with the introduction of the National Service Frameworks and the National Institute of Clinical Excellence (NICE), new targets have been introduced based on clinical evidence. Rigid professional interests and demarcations are slowly giving way to improved interprofessional working practices. Paternalism and dictating to patients what was best for them is changing to providing information and choice. There is now an effort to improve access to services for all, and an attempt to focus on upgrading priority services such as cancer, coronary heart disease, mental health, care of older people, the health of children and the reduction in drug abuse. At the same time, outcomes are being set to maintain existing initiatives and ensure greater patient safety and the clinical governance agenda. The emphasis is on patients and more public involvement with local services.

New systems of monitoring standards and government targets have been introduced that vary from trust boards and local auditing committees to patient watchdogs and the Commission for Health Audit Inspection (CHAI). The latter reviews the implementation of National Service Frameworks (NSFs), such as that for cancer care, at both national and local levels, in relation to clinical governance. Its aims are to review and monitor the implementation of the totality of the clinical governance agenda, and to provide a resource to support healthcare providers in the development of clinical governance (Bishop & Scott 2002). The term 'clinical governance' means the direction and control of the clinical actions, clinical affairs, policies and clinical outcomes that underpin the functioning and purpose of an NHS facility. It represents a deliberate change in direction that places the patient at the heart of the service and encourages health professionals to critically examine their practice in the light of patient needs.

Clinical governance provides an opportunity for advanced nurse practitioners to reflect on ways that they can not only shape the future of nursing care, but also influence the political health agenda and national policy by

- Providing direct nursing care
- Educating, coaching or training patients, families, the public, colleagues and other professionals
- Collaborating, coordinating and playing a significant part in organising the healthcare teams
- Developing protocols, standards, policies and guidelines, to improve quality and health outcomes
- Evaluating, auditing and participating in research
- Providing essential patient/client/family support whenever needed
- Performing tasks, procedures and elements of medicine in a knowledgeable and effective way from a nursing perspective (Castledine 2002).

From a political point of view, these activities place advanced nurses in prime positions to influence the future of healthcare and the political agenda. The main reasons for this are their closeness to the patient and their key roles in monitoring, measuring, evaluating and managing the delivery of care over the critical periods in the patient's ill health and recovery journey. Strong clinical leadership, assertiveness, decision-making and clinical judgement are essential aspects of the advanced nurses' armoury.

Benner *et al.* (1996) claim that the clinical judgement of expert nurses differs greatly from the usual understanding that has dominated the academic culture for the past 30 years. Specifically they claim that

> the clinical judgement of experienced nurses resembles much more the engaged, practical reasoning first described by Aristotle. Experienced nurses reach an understanding of a person's experience with an illness, and hence their response to it, not through abstract labelling such as nursing diagnosis, but rather through knowing the particular patient, his typical pattern of responses, his story and the way in which illness has constituted his story, and through advanced clinical knowledge, which is gained from experience with many persons in similar situations. (Benner *et al.* 1996: 1)

It is important that advanced nurses think and reflect about how they make clinical decisions, how they use evidence to inform that process and what techniques and support can enhance their reasoning (Thompson & Dowding 2002).

The advanced practitioner as a political activist

One of the most underdeveloped and neglected sides of an advanced practitioner's armoury is scholarship and political activism. Much of an advanced practitioner's expertise is developed from technical skills and experience of the patient's specialist health needs. It is important, however, that knowledge is not restricted to medical information and specialist data that does not have a nursing link. Becoming an advanced nurse practitioner differs from expert and specialist nursing practice. It involves not only key tasks but also a more scholarly approach to the patient, their significant others and the whole context in which healthcare is being delivered. Advanced practitioners use all ways of knowing gained from the whole of experience to inform practice. They are working at the boundaries of the profession and should have a vision and flexibility that adapts and considers new possibilities for improving and developing nursing care.

Becoming scholarly helps the practitioner to develop a broad and reflective approach. It is linked to intellectual ability, persistency, independence, integrity and self-discipline. Out of this comes the need to put forward proposals for improving patients' nursing care and advocate for them in the political arena. The professional activist nurse is not one who just happens to be concerned and not one who happens to be a change agent, but one who considers themself a professional agent of change.

The advanced practitioner can develop political awareness by using computer technology to gain access to information. This is especially helpful for practitioners in remote or isolated areas. Staying abreast of changes in policy and regulation through the myriad of available websites is one way of keeping up to date. The quality of website information and the accessibility of web-based links have improved markedly over the past few years, and are set to continue to new heights of information exchange and communication.

Taking part in professional groups and encouraging local interest are ways of developing political understanding. For example, at present there is a need for advanced practitioners to get together and share their experiences. Some of the acknowledged professional organisations, for example, the Royal College of Nursing, are always looking for ideas for conferences and study days. There are also a number of specialist interest groups who want to develop their knowledge and support of nurses working in advanced practice.

Issues for the future

There is no doubt that there are going to be more opportunities for nurses to work in advanced practice. Future roles will require practitioners to work across institutions and settings, following persons with healthcare problems regardless of their location.

This will have implications for the future education of nurses and will require a sound understanding of the complex factors at play in the diverse environments in which practice will take place. One key factor is that of power. Advanced nurses will need to become adept at identifying different sources of power and familiarise themselves with the climate and mechanisms by which it is exercised.

There is also a need to increase the data about advanced nurse practitioners working in the UK. Demographic and outcomes data are sorely lacking on the numbers, mix, geographical location, scope of practice, and patient satisfaction with the service provided. It is important that as many nurses as possible working in these roles not only write up their experiences but also participate in quality initiatives and auditing of their services. The public in particular will continue to experience confusion about the distinctness of the role of the advanced practitioner. Therefore, it is important that all practitioners work closely with their patients and clients, informing them of what is going on.

Currently, the approach in healthcare in the UK is for all providers, including and especially doctors, to be more collaborative and work as a team to integrate care. The advanced practitioner has a key role in encouraging this approach and at times coordinating and ensuring that such collaboration takes place. Significant strides have been made by the present government to pay advanced practitioners at a higher level then ever before. The problem for many of these nurses will be to convince their senior managers that they are worth the money. Therefore, many nurses will have to develop their skills of evaluation, data collection, report-writing and presentation in order to do this. There is no doubt that a career structure is badly needed in which the advanced practitioner can see their possible future clearly mapped out and the criteria and competences for the role clearly articulated.

Conclusion

This chapter has highlighted the importance of the political context of the advanced practitioner's role. It has traced the development of political activism in healthcare over the past few centuries and brought the reader up to date with the political agenda in the UK today. In the early days of the development of the profession there were significant leaders who emerged to take the profession forward. These pioneers often got into trouble and caused much debate and discussion. They stuck to their principles, and their vision and ideas came through. It is important that advanced nurse practitioners develop their political awareness and skills to deal with today's key issues.

With ever increasing demands being made on the nursing profession, it may seem too idealistic and unnecessary to burden nurses with political awareness and responsibilities. However, it is essential to the advanced nurses' role to take up and not only challenge political decisions, but also play an important part in influencing policies. By building and expanding efforts to influence public health policy, nurses will ensure that the practice of nursing does not become a marginalised, invisible part of the NHS. This commitment is not an easy one and involves nurses being aware not only of the health policy and strategy of the current government in power but also of the complex processes required to achieve participation and influence in the wider political arena. It is anticipated that a common understanding will emerge from both the public and healthcare policy-makers regarding advanced nursing's contribution to decreasing costs, increasing access, patient information and participation and the overall quality of healthcare in the UK.

The role of the voluntary sector, nursing organisations, public involvement and regulation are essential to the political healthcare agenda. When this is further influenced by advanced nurse practitioners who are skilled in their own use of evidence-based practice and clinical decision-making, the future political agenda for nursing looks very bright indeed.

One of the easiest ways to encourage nurses to be involved in the political agenda is to critically examine an aspect of NHS policy that is in existence today. There is no better time than the present to begin to identify what is and what is not working well in the emerging new modernised health service. It is up to nurses themselves to take up these opportunities and determine a positive and preferred future for consumers of healthcare, as well as the rest of the nursing profession.

? Key questions for Chapter 16

(1) What is the role of charities in providing healthcare in relation to your field of practice?
(2) What have been some of the key factors in the political realisation of the nursing profession?
(3) What are the arguments for and against the regulation of advanced nursing practice?
(4) What are the key initiatives that an advanced nurse practitioner in your field can take to become more politically aware?

References

Abel-Smith, B. (1960) *History of the Nursing Profession*. London: Heinemann.

American Journal of Nursing, (1908) Editorial. Progress and reaction. *American Journal of Nursing*, 8 (11): 333–4.

Benner, P., Tanner, C.A. & Chesla, C.A. (1996) *Expertise in Nursing Practice: Caring, Clinical Judgement and Ethics*. New York: Springer.

Bishop, V. & Scott, I. (2002) *Challenges in Clinical Practice*. Basingstoke: Palgrave.

Bowman, G. (1967) *The Lamp and the Book: The story of the RCN 1916–1966*. London: The Queen Anne Press.

Castledine, G. (2002) The important aspects of nurse specialist roles. *British Journal of Nursing*, 11 (5): 350.

Daltrop, A. (1978) *Charities* (Past into present series). London: Batsford.

Davies, C. & Beach, A. (2000) *Interpreting Professional Self-regulation: A history of the United Kingdom Central Council for Nursing, Midwifery and Health Visiting*. London: Routledge.

Hutcherson, C. (2002) Role of state boards of nursing in policy. In: *Policy and Politics in Nursing and Health Care*, 4th edn, (eds D.J. Mason, J.K. Leavitt & M.W. Chaffee), pp. 510–13. St Louis: W.B. Saunders.

Lewenson, S.B. (2002) Pride in our past: nursing's political roots. In: *Policy and Politics in Nursing and Health Care*, 4th edn (eds D.J. Mason, J.K. Leavitt & M.W. Chaffee), pp 19–30. St Louis: W.B. Saunders.

Maggs, C.J. (1983) *The Origins of General Nursing*. London: Croom Helm.

Mason. D.J., Leavitt, J.K. & Chaffee, M.W. (2002) *Policy and Politics in Nursing and Health Care*, 4th edn. St Louis. W.B. Saunders.

RCN (1975) *New Horizons in Clinical Nursing. Report of a Seminar held at Leeds Castle, Kent, 14–17 October*. London: RCN.

Reverby, S. (1987) *Order to Care: The Dilemma of American Nursing*. New York: Cambridge University Press.

Scott, H. (2002) Editorial. Government offers nurses 'strings attached' pay awards. *British Journal of Nursing*, 11 (22): 1424.

Thompson, C. & Dowding, D. (2002) *Clinical Decision Making and Judgement in Nursing*. Edinburgh: Churchill Livingstone.

UKCC (2002) *Report of the Higher Level of Practice Pilot and Project*. London: UKCC.

Vance, C., Talbot, S.W., McBride, A. & Mason, D.J. (1985) Coming of age: the women's movement and nursing. In: *Political Action Handbook for Nurses* (eds D. Mason & S Talbot). Menlo Park, CA: Addision-Wesley.

WHO (2000) *Global Advisory Group on Nursing and Midwifery. Report of the 6th Meeting*. Geneva: WHO. Available at www.who.org.

Chapter 17

The Development of a Career Pathway for Advanced Practitioners

George Castledine and Trish Mason

Introduction

Advanced practice represents a major step in the development of nursing in formally providing scope for a considerable degree of autonomous practice. Nurses working at this level can be seen as champions of the growing independence of the profession made possible through a combination of societal and policy changes that have created new opportunities in practice and appropriate educational support. Nurses who have undertaken the additional study required for advanced practice and applied their learning in pioneering new developments are quite rightly seeking rewards for their efforts. In doing so they have drawn attention to the continued lack of a formal, coherent career structure in nursing, the effect of which is to limit opportunities and prospects, especially for those who wish to apply their expertise to direct patient care. Thus nurses reach a particular level of expertise and see no recognisable way forward, no pathway that others have used, so each forges their own route. Whilst this may be productive and enjoyable for individuals, the haphazard nature of this type of career development is very difficult to sell to prospective recruits and offers little certainty to those embarking on nursing careers.

The need for clear career pathways in nursing is not new. This chapter begins with an overview of previous efforts to address the issue, beginning with the Salmon

Report in the 1960s and ending with the proposals set out in the nursing strategy published by the Department of Health (DoH 1999). This is followed by consideration of the current health policy, with particular reference to proposals for the modernisation of the pay system for nurses with associated changes in the career pathways. As yet no firm decisions have been made, but this chapter presents an account of the efforts of two NHS trusts to examine the issues involved and to propose a way forward. The chapter concludes with recommendations for a career pathway for advanced practitioners and presents some key questions for further discussion.

Career pathways in nursing

The Salmon Report (Salmon 1966) was the first real attempt to develop a career ladder for nurses in the UK. The report identified a lot of confusion about the indiscriminate and imprecise use of the title 'matron'. For example, it was applied equally to the nursing heads of large hospitals of over 1000 beds and to those of small hospitals of as few as 10. The only recognition of difference lay in the Whitley salary grading which was based upon the number of beds and not upon the importance of the decisions taken. Assistant or deputy matrons in large hospitals may well have had more onerous tasks than the matron of a small hospital.

Salmon (1966) also identified confusion about the function of nurse administrators in the hospital organisation. Some had management-style roles combined with clinical duties whereas others were solely management- or office-based. Individual matrons tended to hold on to certain clinical or administrative tasks because they enjoyed them even though some could easily have been carried out by a well-trained clerk or more expert clinical nurses who were closer to the patients. It seemed to Salmon that few matrons appeared to practise delegation. Many ward sisters saw the assistant matron as an administrative stepping-stone that was of no great importance or consequence in reaching the matron.

Salmon argued that the nursing career ladder in those days was very narrow and insufficiently developed. Promotion beyond the level of ward sister was severely limited, and there was little incentive for highly competent nurses to stay in the profession. As a way of addressing this, Salmon developed a system of nursing posts grouped and numbered in grades from 10 for the most senior nurse in top management, to 5 for the staff nurse on the ward. Ward sisters and charge nurses provided first-line management, nursing officers and senior nursing officers provided middle management, and principal nursing officers and chief nursing officers filled the most senior levels.

Salmon acknowledged that there were many nurses who did not wish to exchange their expertise in clinical nursing for managerial posts. It was believed, however, that they could still be fitted into the system as nursing officers and senior nursing officers. Salmon argued that the job of the ward sister was physically and mentally demanding, causing many to give up their jobs and move into posts in which there was no clinical contact with patients, for example home sisters. It was suggested that this brain drain could be prevented by encouraging some of these expert ward sisters to take on nursing officer roles but maintain clinical input as well as help with the management and personnel side of the hospital. Unfortunately, all these attempts to develop the careers of nurses in clinical practice failed and it became apparent by the late 1970s that a new career ladder outside the Salmon proposals was needed.

The Royal Commission set up to review the NHS found that there was a need to develop a more clinical career structure for nurses (Merrison 1979). Although it was alleged at the time that the Salmon Committee's recommendations had resulted in a marked increase in the number of nurses employed in administration, the Commission argued that the figures did not support this opinion nor did the structure account for the loss of experienced ward sisters. The Commission took the view that more pertinent reasons for this loss were to be found in demographic and social changes, particularly with regard to the expectations of women (Merrison 1979).

The evidence given to the Merrison Commission at the time emphasised the importance of developing a career structure for clinical specialists i.e. clinical nurse specialists that would encourage ward sisters to stay in their posts and would reward and offer higher levels of promotion to senior clinical nurses (Merrison 1979). It was plain to see that in the early 1980s a nurse who wished to continue to specialise in clinical nursing would have suffered financially as there were no clinical career prospects at the ward sister level. In order to emphasise the importance of the need to develop an improved clinical career structure for nurses above that of nursing sister/charge nurse, Merrison (1979) published a table of nursing salary levels in its final report and firmly recommended that a clinical career structure should be based on the staff nurse and ward sister grades, and that their roles should be reviewed and modified in the light of advances in nursing care. Merrison (1979) further pointed out that rigid definitions of nursing were not helpful and that nurses should be encouraged by both the profession and the Department of Health, to experiment in developing new roles and clinical careers. Nothing significant happened, however, following the publication of the report and the first generation of nurse specialists and advanced practitioners developed their roles without any direction or control. There was little evaluation or audit of what was going on, which later led to problems in identifying the characteristics of specialist, advanced and other new roles.

A second generation of specialist and advanced practitioners evolved in the 1990s in the wake of the United Kingdom Central Council's report on post-registration education and practice (UKCC 1994). This report represented an attempt to define what specialist and advanced nurses should be doing but it gave rise to such confusion that the Council later changed tack and identified two levels of practice: specialist and higher-level (UKCC 2002).

In the late 1990s a new Labour government sought to encourage major role developments in nursing and expansion towards advanced practice as part of its modernisation programme. The White Papers *The New NHS: Modern, Dependable* (DoH 1997) and, more particularly, *Making a Difference* (DoH 1999) made it clear that the government was committed to developing the nurse's clinical role. *Making a Difference* was an important document for outlining the government's proposed clinical career levels for nurses. It proposed the introduction of nurse consultants capable of working at advanced practice level and earning the highest salaries in clinical nursing. The key to the successful development of nurse consultants still hinges on their differences with regard to existing nurse specialists, their relationship to patients and their value to nursing care. Nurse consultants must be careful that they do not fall into the trap of being used as substitutes for medical staff and lose their fundamental nursing competences. Nurse consultants cannot develop from special courses or be expected to appear overnight. The role should be seen as a natural development and progression for some generalist and specialist nurses.

Clinical development structure

It would seem that there are three avenues of clinical development after initial registration as a nurse. The first avenue is open to clinical nurses who want to stay in general nursing practice and not specialise in any way. The second avenue is available to those nurses who wish to specialise or sub-specialise into areas which may be medically led or geared towards specialist nursing competences. The third avenue is a much more restricted entry and may be available only to those nurses who have developed their roles in generalist or more commonly specialist practice. This third avenue is, therefore, the only one that the UKCC referred to as higher-level practice; other countries refer to it as 'advanced practice'.

A new clinical career structure is set to replace the old clinical grading system (NHS Executive 1999). The government claims that this will provide better career progression and fairer rewards for nurses who develop new skills and expand their roles. However, within each of the three career bands for registered nurses there needs to be further discussion on competences and pay progression scales. These will presumably be aimed at encouraging individual development within one particular band. The government suggests using spine points within each individual band, which could be linked to local competence frameworks developed by employers to recognise and reward innovative and progressive team players. The key to the successful development of nurse consultants, and thus advanced practitioners, may then hinge on how they relate not only to their patients but also to the rest of the nursing and healthcare team. The consultant role in nursing should be about sharing and developing clinical nursing. The main skill of consultant nurses must be the ability to communicate easily and effectively with all those concerned with the patients'/clients' healthcare. It is to be hoped that postholders will bring to the consultant role a more humane, personal and caring approach than has ever been seen at this level of professional hierarchy. No one particular course can achieve this as it takes a certain personality with experience and an ability to apply knowledge and make meaningful relationships throughout the various proposed career bands.

Those nurses who have striven, sometimes under great financial and personal pressures, to develop their education and competences will welcome the new proposals. However, given nursing's obsession with hierarchy, status and medicalisation, it is to be hoped that practitioners will not just concentrate on developing medical skills that are far removed from practical nursing. In addition, the proposals suggest that the new career structure will provide better opportunities to combine or move laterally between jobs in practice, education and research. It is to be hoped that this will mean the development of more joint appointments and closer links with higher education in nursing. If not, there is a danger that nurse clinicians' pay will surge ahead of nurse lecturers' pay, thus dissuading future expert nurses from going into education and research. Finally, the proposals include the reintroduction of a nursing cadet system that will offer individuals a vocational route into nursing that would allow them to progress all the way to consultant. In some parts of the UK, entry onto some nursing courses is considered extremely difficult as universities demand too high an academic level. Therefore, it will be interesting to see how many of these schemes develop and the proportion of nurses entering the profession in this way.

Higher-level practice

The publication of the final report of the UKCC's higher-level practice project confirmed the view that there were two levels of practice beyond the point of initial registration: specialist and advanced practice (UKCC 2002). Explicit standards in the form of learning outcomes were set for specialist practice and a conceptual descriptor of advanced practice was offered. However, because of the rapid changes that occurred in healthcare practice, such as the significant increase in specialist nurses, the UKCC decided to re-examine its post-registration framework and the levels of practice. The UKCC, therefore, established a group that explored what was envisaged as the upper levels of nursing and midwifery practice. A draft descriptor, standard and assessment system was produced and tested with users, the profession and stakeholders across the UK. This resulted in what the UKCC referred to as the development of a standard, which identified specific outcomes against which practitioners could be assessed, and the design of an assessment system.

The standard was laid out under seven broad headings: providing effective healthcare; improving quality and health outcomes; evaluation and research; leading and developing practice; innovation and changing practice; developing the self and others; and working across professional and organisational boundaries. The standard and assessment system were piloted by City & Guilds Affinity in order to list the standard as a basis of assessing fitness to practice at the higher level, and indicated that the majority of participants expressed positive views about the standard and the extent to which it was relevant and achievable. This pilot has contributed to the consultant nurse/midwife/health visitor initiatives in the UK and is being used by employers to structure job descriptions, inform lifelong learning and to support risk management strategies. The UKCC's work has been shared with representatives of other regulatory bodies, professional organisations and trade unions, and employers of other health and social care professions. Following the pilot, the UKCC has refined the higher-level practice standard and the revised version is in the report. Improving the guidance and producing a system design manual have enhanced the validity and reliability of the assessment process.

The Shrewsbury and Telford hospitals study

Research at Shrewsbury and Telford hospitals resulted in a very positive approach to recognising and helping nurses develop their careers in advanced nursing practice.

The research clearly lays out the stages of clinical specialisation and competence development, and shows what can be achieved if there is appropriate and adequate management support. The senior nursing management team at both the Royal Shrewsbury Hospital and the Princess Royal Hospital in Telford were keen to help identify where their senior and specialist nursing practitioners stood in relation to all the proposed developments coming from the government, the UKCC and the profession. There was a firm and positive commitment to developing staff and helping them realise their career aspirations and potential for advanced nursing practice.

The study consisted of interviewing and reviewing all the nurse specialists in both hospitals. Although some members of the clinical staff were suspicious and anxious about the process, it soon became clear that the aim of the study was to help them and was not a regrading exercise. In fact, many of the specialist nurses found the exercise helpful in clarifying where they were in their careers and what aspects of their role still needed further development.

The UKCC's work on higher-level practice and, in particular, the descriptor and standard of the seven areas of competence were used at the two hospitals to clarify the differences between nurse specialists' roles and those of advanced nurses or nurse consultants. The findings showed that nurse specialists spent the majority of their time in clinical practice and consultation, with 25% of time being spent in education and scholarly activities, although this varied from one individual to another. Many nurse specialists were developing strategies to modify practice requirements and cost-effective innovations in delivery systems, thus enhancing quality patient care. The majority were developing their knowledge base. There was much confusion about the actual role and responsibilities of the nurse specialist, with members of various healthcare professions, particularly doctors, holding different expectations of the nurse specialist role.

The research confirmed that nurse specialists and advanced practitioners improve access to care, competently manage care for patients in a variety of healthcare settings, are extremely well accepted by patients, and provide high-quality care. Many of the nurse specialists and advanced practitioners felt isolated and cut off from their nursing colleagues. Sometimes it was difficult for them to keep up to date with the general professional nursing issues. It was therefore recommended that all of them would benefit by closer networking and management by a senior nurse manager who took an active interest in their work and development. In addition, they needed to be more thoroughly integrated into the organisation by various means and required to produce an annual report of their activities that included a review of how they had met their objectives and patient outcomes.

The pioneers of nurse specialisation have focused their energies, creativity and determination on chiselling out roles to deliver their unique and important contributions to patient care. However, the healthcare landscape is changing rapidly and there is an urgent need for all nurse specialists to make sure that they are in tune with the wider organisation in which they work. The measurement of outcomes has become an important component of evaluating healthcare and it was recommended that nurse specialists see themselves as part of this outcomes model. This is particularly important because, as nurse specialists and advanced practitioners have traditionally been involved in unique and diverse aspects of patient-focused care, outcomes measurements can now enable the significant contributions of nurse specialists to be realised.

The findings demonstrated the evolution of several domains of nurse specialist and advanced practice:

- Help with diagnostic/patient monitoring
- Management of patients' health/illness
- Counselling and being available
- Coordinating and helping to clarify in simple, straightforward language the patients' problems and needs
- Administering/monitoring therapeutic interventions and regimes
- Monitoring/ensuring quality of healthcare practices
- Teaching/coaching role
- Consulting
- Scholarly activities, research and publications
- Advanced assessment skills and competences in a variety of medical procedures.

The degree to which individuals accomplish these roles depends on their knowledge and experience. As they become more expert in their field they may well add to or modify these aspects. Many nurse specialist and advanced practitioners' roles seem to be centred on medical diagnosis, treatment or patient-monitoring functions. This is probably because many specialist nursing and advanced practice roles began as medical initiatives and doctors are confident only when referring to the medical aspects of the nurse specialist and advanced practice work. There is a danger that the nurse specialist and advanced practitioner may follow only the medicalised descriptor of their role because of the lack of national nursing directives and the failure of the nursing profession to define not only specialist nursing and advanced nursing practice, but also essential nursing practice. Consequently, the research attempted to clarify what it is about specialist and advanced nursing roles that identified them as unique and of value to not only medicine but also nursing. The answer lay in the response of patients and their significant others in relation to what they felt was important about the nurse specialist and advanced practitioner.

From a medical perspective, the value of the nurse specialist and advanced practitioner was that they gained vital specialist information that fed into the patient's medical records. The nurse specialist/advanced practitioner might also be performing a key coordinating role in that junior doctors come and go but the nurse specialist and advanced practitioner was always there to fill the gaps and maintain the continuity of the medical service. Another medical advantage of nurse specialist and advanced practitioner's work was that they became expert in the medical treatment of the patient and developed strict protocols and guidelines. Patients and doctors liked this approach because they felt confident that if the nurse noticed something different or significant, they would refer the patient immediately to the consultant for an expert opinion. In addition, scarce medical resources could be diverted to more complex and difficult cases.

The nursing aspects of the role centred on being available and supportive at the right time and place for the patient. Having a nurse to talk to and to interpret what the doctors have said, was crucial. The nurse specialist and advanced practitioner were both skilled in assessment techniques and were able to pick up patients' associated physical and psychological problems. Nurse specialists and advanced practitioners were also a fount of expert knowledge and support for not only their patients, but also their nursing colleagues. It was their nursing responsibility to pass on to others as much information and knowledge as they could.

Key factors relating to specialist and advanced nurses

The Shrewsbury and Telford hospital studies and work by Castledine in other NHS hospital trusts demonstrated that:

- Specialist nurses and advanced practitioners are isolated
- They should all be participating in clinical supervision that may be provided by medical doctors or senior nursing colleagues, depending on the local situation
- There are two levels or avenues of specialist nurse and advanced practitioner development with the majority of nurses fitting into specialist practice and only one or two nurses working in a higher level in many hospital trusts
- There are several stages in the career pathway from nurse specialist to advanced practitioner, with not all nurse specialists becoming advanced nurse practitioners (Fig. 17.1).

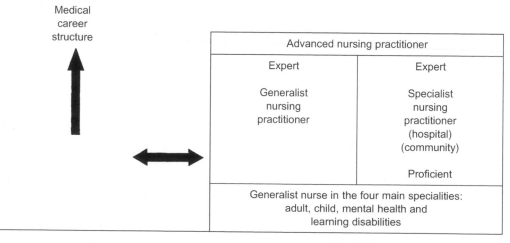

Fig. 17.1 The routes of a clinical nursing career structure. The proposed clinical career structure emphasises 'nursing' in the practitioner's title; outside this is the nurse practitioner who wishes to develop a more medical focus or bias in their work.

Key factors in clinical practice

The following domains of specialist practice are applicable to all and should be used as a base to describe the content of each nurse specialist and advanced practitioner's role.

- Use a variety of assessment techniques, not necessarily used by nurses before, to elicit patient information regarding their specialist nursing needs and total patient care.
- Help with diagnosing and monitoring medical and nursing information.
- Play a key role in the management of the patient's journey through the illness, disability, rehabilitation and adjustment experience.
- Coordinate care where required, clarifying and communicating patient information in a simple, straightforward language, appropriate to the patient and significant others' needs.
- Be there when the patient needs help, counselling and supporting where appropriate.
- Develop a variety of competences in medical procedures without detriment to core nursing values and principles.
- Administer and monitor a variety of specialist therapeutic interventions and regimes. Set standards in collaboration with other healthcare professionals.
- Teach and coach the patient and significant others in a way that promotes skill enhancement, independence, self-care and education.
- Monitor and evaluate self and others' contribution to care, using a variety of tools and techniques.
- Participate in scholarly activities such as research, academic presentations and publications so that patient care is improved and nursing knowledge is promoted and developed.

Recommendations for clinical practice

- In order to develop their role, some nurse specialists would benefit from an advanced nursing assessment skills course. This should be linked with their individual appraisal and discussed with their manager.
- Nurse specialists and advanced practitioners should be more proactive in promoting their role and educating other nursing colleagues so that they do not de-skill them and mislead nurses into thinking that they should wait until the nurse specialist arrives before doing anything.
- Some nurse specialists and advanced practitioners are maintaining their own nursing record systems. Often these are kept in their own offices or places of work. Such systems should be integrated into the patient's own hospital record as there is a risk of gaps in communication and leaks in confidentiality. Where nurse specialists are writing and keeping nursing records, these should be carefully reviewed, monitored and discussed.

- One of the key competences of a nurse specialist and advanced practitioner is that they should be excellent communicators and coordinators of care. All nurse specialists and advanced practitioners should carefully review this aspect of their work.
- All nurse specialists and advanced practitioners should be evaluating their practice through audit and other relevant methods.
- All nurse specialists and advanced practitioners should be exploring ways to investigate the core nursing commonalities between their different roles and ways to enhance the uniqueness of the nursing contribution.

Recommendations for management

- Nurse specialists and advanced practitioners need to develop professional networks with other nurse specialist and advanced practitioners to gain peer support and professional development.
- Nurse specialists and advanced practitioners should be well supported by a management system that prevents them from becoming isolated.
- Local regulation of their activities should be carried out to protect both them and the patients they care for.
- All nurse specialists and advanced practitioners should produce an annual report containing audits and outcomes of their work.
- Secretarial and administrative support should be reviewed.
- Progressive planning and replacement of senior nurse specialists and advanced practitioners should be considered, with opportunities created for junior nursing staff.
- Annual review should be encouraged to update and keep senior management informed of developments in nurse specialist and advanced practitioner roles.
- To avoid confusion, all nurse specialists should use one title, except those appointed as nurse consultants. The title that should be used is: nurse specialist (speciality).
- The progression of nurse specialists should follow the seven stages of the Castledine model (Table 17.1).
- Nurse specialists and advanced practitioners should be paid according to their assessed position on the Castledine model.
- The trust should regularly update its directory of nurse specialists and advanced practitioners.

Recommendations for education

- Nurse specialists and advanced practitioners should be very careful with regard to the types of course they follow. The courses should be aimed at developing their role and justified on the basis of their value to future patient care.
- Mentorship should be encouraged and a variety of methods considered.
- All nurse specialists and advanced practitioners should be developing a specialist/

Table 17.1 Castledine's stages of career development.

Stages	Achievements
1	General nurse working in a speciality General nurse with some experience, competence and education in the speciality
2	General nurse proceeding at early beginner stage to become a recognised nurse specialist in a defined specialist area
3	General nurse developing into a nurse specialist
4	Recognition as a nurse specialist
5	Refining work as an expert nurse specialist and/or moving to advanced specialist nursing
6	Recognised as an advanced nurse practitioner
7	Expert advanced nurse practitioner developing/adding to experience, knowledge and competence

advanced nurse profile, detailing their clinical supervision, personal development and education.

Conclusion

The development of a clinical career structure for nurses working in specialist and advanced practice goes back to recommendations made in the Merrison Report in 1979. There has always been a desire to develop a method for expert clinical nurses to achieve status and economic advancement without leaving the bedside or the interface with patients. It has taken over 20 years to achieve clarification and recognition of what it is that specialist and advanced clinical nurses do.

Following work by the UKCC (1994) on the standards for post-registration education and practice, it became clear that specialist and advanced practitioners exercise higher levels of judgement, discretion and decision-making in clinical care. They are able to monitor and improve standards of care through supervision of practice, clinical audit, the provision of skilled professional leadership, and the development of practice through research, teaching and the support of professional colleagues.

Figure 17.1 shows three main routes that a registered nurse can follow to stay in clinical practice: specialist nursing role moving onto advanced practice, stay in general nursing and then move into advanced practice. Nurses wishing to follow a more technical, medical approach to their work can become paramedical nurse practitioners, move into medical practice and follow a medical career.

Following studies carried out in several hospital trusts, particularly those in Shrewsbury and Telford, it has now become possible to identify and clarify where all specialist nurses are in relation to their position and development on clinical career pathways such as the Castledine model. Clinical experience, specialist higher-level competences, education, recognition and contribution to interdisciplinary care are crucial factors in this process. Concern for specialist and advanced practitioners is an important form of support that should be expressed explicitly rather than assumed.

Many of the specialist and advanced practitioners' career goals can be advanced within the context of the organisation. The Shrewsbury and Telford hospitals study has shown that career planning can benefit both the organisation and the individual, and this model can be used to identify the elements of a career development process for future nurses wishing to stay in clinical practice.

 Key questions for Chapter 17

(1) What support could be provided by employers of advanced nurse practitioners in your field of practice?
(2) What are some of the commonalities of specialist and advanced practitioners in their career development?
(3) To what extent is the Castledine model helpful in evaluating your career to date?
(4) To what extent can the recommendations made in this chapter be applied in your work setting?

References

DoH (1997) *The New NHS. Modern: Dependable*. London: DoH.

DoH (1999) *Making a Difference: Strengthening the Nursing, Midwifery and Health Visiting Contribution to Health and Healthcare*. London: DoH.

Merrison Report (1979) *Royal Commission on the National Health Service*, Chairman Sir A. Merrison. London: HMSO.

NHS Executive (1999) *Agenda for Change: Modernising the NHS Pay System. Joint Framework of Principles and Agreed Statement on the Way Forward*, Health Service Circular 1999/227. Available at http://www.doh.gov.uk

Salmon (1966) *Report of the Committee on Senior Nursing Staff Structure*. London: HMSO.

UKCC (1994) *The Standards for Post-registration Education and Practice Project*. London: UKCC.

UKCC (2002) *The Executive Summary of the Higher Level Practice Project*. London: UKCC.

Chapter 18

Future Directions in Advanced Nursing Practice in the UK

Paula McGee and George Castledine

Introduction

In the previous edition of this book we put forward our ideas and concerns about the future of advanced practice. We argued that, historically, developments in nursing roles took place alongside increased specialisation in medicine. We emphasised the need for new and emergent nursing roles to retain their professional identity and avoid overreliance on the medical model or its associated technology. We took the view that advanced practice must retain at its core a focus on and commitment to nursing and examine new ways of expressing nursing values and skills in patient care. Since then, the UKCC project on higher-level practice has explored ways in which this focus and commitment can be achieved and demonstrated through an identified and tested standard for practice (UKCC 2002). The Department of Health has addressed the issue of new, including advanced, nursing roles and identified ways in which experienced and knowledgeable practitioners may enhance their contribution to a reformed NHS by providing leadership in nursing and in service delivery (DoH 1999, 2000, 2001). The DoH has also recognised the need for a career structure in nursing that accommodates such roles, proposing three levels of practice and creating the possibility of higher salaries for the most senior nurses who remained in practice.

In this book we have presented our most recent ideas about advanced practice for nursing in the UK. We have proposed that advanced practice is a state of professional maturity in which the individual demonstrates a level of integrated knowledge, skill and competence that challenges the accepted boundaries of practice and pioneers developments in healthcare. We have argued that professional maturity is achieved through a synthesis of experience and formal study that equip the individual to adopt a critical approach to practice through which the boundaries of nursing are examined and tested for the benefit of patients. The advanced practitioner is able to draw on scholarly, interpersonal and reflective skills to envision challenges to the status quo and initiate new possibilities for nursing that both contribute directly to the enhancement of patient care and lead others to do the same. Contributors to this book have examined various aspects of our view of the advanced role, taking into account the nature of nursing practice in the UK, particularly with regard to advanced health assessment, current health policy, ways of determining competence and benchmarking.

Advanced nursing practice is now a global phenomenon, with over 30 countries either developing or exploring roles that serve to broaden access to healthcare. The International Council of Nurses has provided a broad definition of this level of nursing that reflects the complex knowledge and skill required whilst leaving individual states free to determine how these may be applied to meet the specific needs of their populations (ICN 2002). Each country, including the UK, faces its own challenges in providing healthcare and it is likely that advanced roles will develop in unique ways whilst conforming to internationally agreed criteria, for example about the authority to diagnose and initiate treatment.

It is apparent, from the experiences of nurses in those countries in which advanced roles have been introduced, that establishing such authority and acquiring the clinical expertise needed to exercise it can challenge not only accepted practice in nursing but also traditional relationships with other professions, most notably medicine. Contributors to this book have, therefore, examined some of these challenges within the context of the UK and presented examples and ideas for future development of advanced roles based on interprofessional cooperation.

Throughout this book we have emphasised the importance of further exploration, prompted by key questions on the topics discussed in each chapter. This final chapter begins by revisiting those key questions, drawing on them to create an agenda for research into advanced practice that we hope will inform future investigations. This agenda has a strong focus on practice but also takes into account the need to evaluate the impact of advanced practice in relation to health policy and multidisciplinary working. We then consider two additional matters: the implications of the proposed reforms of the pay system in the NHS and the impact of first contact services in the community in terms of their significance for advanced practice. We present our recommendations in relation to these issues followed by our ideas for advanced practice in the future and the ways in which we see the role continuing to develop.

An agenda for research

At the end of each chapter in this book (with the exception of Chapter 15) we have presented a list of key questions in which readers have been asked to consider specific issues in relation their own fields of practice or work settings. The purpose of these questions is to promote further discussion as a basis for investigation into the realities of implementing the advanced practice role. In our view, the topics covered by these questions can be grouped into nine themes.

(1) Clinical practice

We take the view that practice is paramount in advanced practice. The advanced practitioner must possess and be able to apply an extensive repertoire of relevant clinical expertise. This application requires advanced practitioners to spend a significant proportion of their time engaged in direct care activities that may range from total care of a patient, particularly those with complex or unusual needs, and working with staff to help them develop new skills, to intervening in a crisis (Koetters 1989). We support Hamric's (2000: 60) argument that 'the reason the profession exists is to render nursing services to individuals in need of them'. Nursing management, education and other fields provide well-established senior roles in which some advanced skills are essential but these are not used in the provision of direct care to patients. If advanced practitioners are to fulfil the role outlined by the ICN (2002), then direct clinical practice is an essential part of their role. There is no point in acquiring the level of knowledge and skill required unless it is applied to directly to patients. However, the nature of direct care activities requires further exploration and we particularly recommend research that clarifies the contributions that advanced practitioners can make towards improving patient outcomes and satisfaction, the skills and confidence of staff, and the overall quality of nursing care.

(2) Evidence-based practice

The advanced practitioner can bring about improvements in patient care by promoting and contributing to evidence-based practice. This is the 'conscientious, explicit and judicious use of current best evidence in making decisions about the care of individual patients' (Sackett *et al.* 1996). This evidence may be the outcome of research, audit, expert opinion, patient views or a combination of all of these.

The advanced practitioner requires first the ability to evaluate evidence, selecting the most robust elements and assessing the applicability of these to both the field of practice and the particular work setting. Having selected appropriate evidence, the advanced practitioner requires the skills needed to work with staff in testing and applying the evidence to patient care. Alternatively, if the evidence available is insufficient or unsatisfactory then the advanced practitioner should be able to generate questions for research and either undertake systematic investigations as a member of a research team or facilitate others to do so. Finally, the advanced practitioner requires the ability to disseminate the outcomes of such investigations through written reports, conference presentations and published work that provide opportunities for others to benefit from the outcomes.

We take the view that many aspects of nursing, particularly those activities that are referred to as 'basic nursing care', have received limited attention from researchers. Moreover, the constantly changing and complex nature of healthcare places new, unexplored demands on staff. Advanced practitioners' involvement in direct care activities means that they are ideally placed to identify topics for research that can be of direct benefit to patients and staff at local level. We therefore recommend that advanced practitioners develop the skills required for research and utilise these in both promoting evidence-based practice and furthering nursing knowledge.

(3) *Diversity and inclusiveness*

Access to healthcare is a universal human right regardless of an individual's characteristics that may, in social contexts, contribute to marginalisation or exclusion. In the UK, the right of everyone to healthcare is evident in current health policy that emphasises commitment to the NHS as a service that is available to the whole population based on clinical need and free at the point of delivery. The right to healthcare is also evident in the nurses' professional code of practice that explicitly prohibits discrimination against any patient on the grounds of sex, race, religion, culture, sexual orientation or any other factor. We fully support this move towards inclusiveness and the efforts made throughout the NHS to ensure a more equitable provision of services. However, we also take the view that there is still much to be done, particularly at local levels, in challenging entrenched attitudes and practices and in creating services that move beyond window-dressing to truly meet the needs of diverse subsections of the population.

In Chapter 11 we have argued the case for cultural competence as a key component in advanced practice. We see that competence directed towards improvements in care for patients who are members of black or minority ethnic groups. In Chapter 3 we argued that the culturally-competent advanced practitioner is one who has a sound grasp of the culture of the organisation, who has power and authority, and who understands the relationships between staff and managers, the rituals and traditions that punctuate working life and the degree to which the organisation welcomes change. In both those chapters we proposed that cultural competence was an evolving state dependent on a combination of self-awareness, interpersonal skills, knowledge and exposure to cultures that informed the adaptation of practice and the development of new ways of working.

Here we argue that those skills should also be applied in meeting the needs of other groups in society. The term 'diversity' applies not only to black and minority ethnic groups but also to others, such as the homeless who are socially excluded, women, who may have less power and freedom than men, and those whose beliefs, values or sexual orientation are stigmatised. The advanced practitioner can apply the same skills to develop self-awareness about personal attitudes and values that might impinge on working with members of particular groups and enable others to do the same. The advanced practitioner can apply research skills in systematically investigating the health problems and needs of specific local groups and use the evidence obtained to develop or adapt services. Finally the advanced practitioner can work with staff, facilitating changes that improve patient care. We recommend that advanced practitioners consider diversity a priority in their work, utilise their research skills to discover the nature of diversity in the local area and establish appropriate evidenced-based practice that truly meets the needs of those concerned.

(4) *Interface with other service providers*

The development of advanced roles challenges the accepted boundaries of practice between nursing and other health professions, particularly medicine. In the USA, advanced practice has engendered considerable hostility among some medical practitioners who feel that their traditional roles are under threat and see new nursing roles as a further encroachment on their territory. As we have shown in Chapter 12, there is evidence of formal, collective opposition to advanced practice. This has not, so far, been the case in the UK, but practitioners in both camps are right to be concerned about the changing nature of their roles and question the ways in which society expects them to apply their particular knowledge and skills. Already there is some evidence of overlap between advanced nursing and medical roles, with each applying the similar knowledge and skill in a different way (Hunsberger *et al.* 1992).

The interface between nursing and medicine has overshadowed the potential for conflict between advanced practice and other health professions. Very little attention has been paid to the impact of advanced practice on, for example, physiotherapist, dietician, pharmacist, podiatrist or any complementary role such as that of acupuncturist. This is a little ironic as some modern health professions have their origins in nursing and in certain fields of practice such as palliative care, nurses have pioneered the inclusion of complementary therapies into mainstream patient care. We therefore recommend research that seeks to address the interface between advanced nursing and all other roles involved in healthcare.

(5) *Professional regulation and control*

A key concern in the development of advanced practice must be that of public protection. This has several dimensions. First, the public must be assured of the competence of nurses undertaking advanced practice roles. In this book we have shown that competence is a concept that eludes a single, agreed definition. Notions of competence are contingent upon competing views of professional roles as viewed from the varying perspectives of individual practitioners, nursing organisations and external groups such as the sector skills council Skills for Health. Inherent in these views are differing ideas on how competence can be made explicit and demonstrated to others. The UKCC's work on higher-level practice has demonstrated one approach to the assessment of competence at an advanced level that appears to be applicable not only across diverse fields of practice but also in each of the four countries of the UK (UKCC 2002). However, further work is needed to apply this assessment systematically and we therefore recommend research that continues to examine the notion of competence in advanced practice.

Second, when this is achieved, the Nursing and Midwifery Council has to find a satisfactory way of recording that individuals have reached the standard required and ensuring that they maintain their fitness to practise at an advanced level. Whilst this sounds very simple, the Council has inherited a complex register of nurses as well as other responsibilities that have traditionally been focused mainly on entry to the profession. Advanced practice is only one of many post-registration roles that must be considered in developing systems of recording and regulation that are effective, easily accessible and economic to maintain.

Third, regardless of which views about competence eventually predominate, effort will be needed to convince the public that advanced practitioners are capable of meeting a substantial part of their health needs without automatic reference to a doctor. This requires a public education campaign that explains advanced roles, emphasises competence and makes clear that advanced practitioners are neither substitutes for doctors nor substandard, second-best healthcare. We therefore recommend research that examines the information needs of the public and contributes to the development of appropriate strategies for education about advanced practice.

(6) *Providing professional leadership*

In this book we have promoted the view that transformational leadership is an essential component of advanced practice. This type of leadership is based on the concept of reciprocity in that the leader clarifies what is to be achieved in terms that inspire others to both follow and actively participate in ways that enable them to fulfil their own goals (Marriner-Tomey 1993). In other words the transformational leader is astute in creating win–win situations in which all parties stand to benefit.

There are three elements in transformational leadership: charisma, valuing individuals and intellectual stimulation. In advanced practice, charisma is part of the personal attributes that enable the practitioner to communicate a vision of what is to be achieved and how it may be done in ways that motivate others to take part in the process. That motivation is dependent on the advanced practitioner's demonstration of respect for others as experienced professionals in their own right who can actively contribute to refining the vision and the means by which it can be achieved. The transformational leader values these contributions, seeks and incorporates into the plan of action the particular knowledge and strengths of individuals. Actively contributing and participating provides a basis for intellectual stimulation that enables followers to identify goals that will benefit them as well as the enterprise being undertaken (Marriner-Tomey 1993). That enterprise is likely to be concerned with bringing about changes in practice that result in improvements to patient care. We take the view that more research is needed to identify examples of sound and effective transformational leadership in practice and ways in which advanced practitioners can best acquire and apply the skills required.

(7) *User views*

There is no doubt that public expectations of services are increasing, particularly with regard to healthcare. Societal changes have created a more questioning challenging population that is no longer content to believe that professionals always know best. Service users, therefore, want to have a say in how the NHS should be run, identifying the services they need and determining how these are delivered. We take the view that the advanced practitioner has a major role to play in building relationships with voluntary organisations related to the specific field of practice for two reasons. First, the advanced practitioner has a commitment to direct patient care and to improving that care through the application of clinical expertise, transformational leadership and evidenced-based practice. Second, the advanced practitioner is interpersonally and culturally competent. The combination of these competences facilitates working with personnel from quite diverse backgrounds, enabling them to make their views known. Inherent in seeking user views and participation are the issues of credibility and trustworthiness. If service users are to be truly involved in the development and delivery of services then they need to feel that professionals value their views and act upon them.

Voluntary organisations may provide the main source of advice and support for patients and are thus in a strong position to work with professionals in bringing about improvements by presenting the major concerns and experiences of members. However, the advanced practitioner must bear in mind that voluntary organisations may have different agendas from those of the public sector. For example, there may be more than one organisation associated with a particular condition, with differing priorities and interests. The advanced practitioner will need to develop ways of listening constructively and evaluating contributions whilst avoiding taking sides. In addition, it may be beneficial to set up local processes through which the views and experiences of the patients and their families who actually use the local services can be canvassed first-hand, and we recommend that advanced practitioners use their research skills to determine the most appropriate ways of enabling service users to make their wishes known and acted upon.

Improved access to information, particularly via the Internet, means that patients can now be as well-informed as professionals. It is no longer unusual for patients to come to clinic clutching pages downloaded from the Net and ask, 'Why am I not having this treatment?' How the practitioner reacts to the well-informed patient is a test of professional maturity. The credibility and trustworthiness of the advanced practitioner are likely to be enhanced by a preparedness to engage with the patient as a knowledgeable equal. Such engagement is all the more important when patients have accessed websites containing material that is inappropriate to their needs, inaccurate or in some cases, harmful. We recommend that advanced practitioners familiarise themselves with the most common sites likely to be accessed by patients in their fields of practice, seek ways to evaluate these and encourage others to do the same (see the exercise at the end of the chapter). We further recommend that advanced practitioners examine ways of providing sound web-based information for patients.

(8) Education

Throughout this book we have emphasised the importance of education in the development of the advanced practitioner, and Chapter 7 has outlined one way in which the necessary competences can be achieved. We see education as a means of facilitating critical practice in which the combined skills of analysis, reflection and evaluation are directed towards a creative but rigorous appraisal of nursing care. However, the level and nature of the education required place great demands not only on the student but also on the tutorial staff. Very little attention has been paid to the developmental needs of tutorial staff in facilitating the development of advanced practitioners, and we therefore recommend programmes of research that address this issue.

(9) Recording developments

In Chapter 2 we presented an outline of the historical development of advanced practice in the UK. Preparing that chapter was like trying to assemble a jigsaw in which many of the pieces were missing because, at the time, no one thought to keep records or write accounts of the events taking place. We therefore recommend that all those involved in advanced practice write accounts or maintain some form of record of developments.

Advanced practice and employment

The NHS Plan introduced an agenda for reform aimed at both improving the accessibility and quality of the services provided to patients and the working conditions for staff. The intention was to create a working environment in which staff felt valued rather than 'rushed off their feet and constantly exhausted; where careers are developed not stagnant; where staff are paid properly for good performance' (DoH 2000: 17). The Plan stated a commitment to increases in staffing based on more places in training schools and a national recruitment campaign, improvements in pay and more general improvements in working lives through the introduction of flexible working practices, better career structures and opportunities for training. Alongside these considerations are the projected workforce requirements that identify the numbers of staff needed to maintain and sustain growth in the health sector and the European Working Time Directive that will reduce doctors' hours to 56 per week in 2004.

Proposals for improvements in pay are intended to simplify and modernise the current system in ways that take account of new practices and responsibilities (NHS Executive 1999). A key element in these proposals is the evaluation of every job based on the

- Knowledge and skills needed to do the work required
- Amount and level of responsibility involved
- Physical, mental or emotional effort required.

These evaluations will, for the most part, take place at local level, although some posts may be reviewed on a national basis to prevent local services becoming overburdened. The intention is to create a new, nationally-based relationship between the requirements of each job and salary. Allied to these factors is a commitment to the development of clearly defined career progression pathways linked to continuous professional development and lifelong learning (NHS Executive 1999). Conditions of service are also to be modernised and simplified, with some degree of local flexibility allowed.

These proposals reflect the need for new ways of working that move away from established patterns of roles and demarcation. Professionals will have to be prepared to hand over some aspects of their work to sections of the workforce that are currently unqualified as a step towards unlocking their potential and providing flexible career routes through which they may progress to professional levels. In this scenario, advanced practitioners can be vulnerable because their jobs are not well-defined. Establishing an advanced post requires a joint investment of time by both the individual practitioner and the managers concerned, to ensure that the interests of both are openly considered and protected.

Shay *et al.* (1996) recommend that this investment is formally constituted under the auspices of a practice agreement committee that includes representatives from nursing, medicine and administration and that takes responsibility for discussing and agreeing practice standards and defining the advanced role in the particular setting. The committee should produce a job description that includes the qualifications and attributes needed to do the job. The committee should also clarify the model of practice to be used, addressing matters such as the scope of practice, authority for initiating referrals and investigations, prescribing, and beginning or altering treatment. Inherent in this clarification is the need to ensure that the employing organisation has the appropriate insurance cover and it may be essential to seek both legal and insurance advice.

Shay *et al.*'s (1996) proposals represent sound advice. Nurses who are developing advanced roles need to ensure that they do so in ways that enable them to use their expertise appropriately in ways that benefit patients. Managers need to make sure that patients are safely cared for and that the advanced practitioner's knowledge and skills are being used to the best advantage. This includes ensuring that the interface with medicine is addressed from the start so that the doctors concerned understand what is involved in the new post. However, setting up a post in this way does not in itself guarantee every eventuality. Advanced practice is still a fairly new concept in the UK and it is often not possible to anticipate all the demands and implications of a post when it is first developed. It is also important that nurses who take advanced practice posts are not disadvantaged financially and that they continue to have access to career progression and professional education.

The NHS Plan introduced an agenda for improvements in working lives. For junior doctors the opportunities included a reduction in their working hours, increased training and the introduction of better career structures (DoH 2000). More recent proposals have expanded on this commitment in addressing the need to reform the senior house officer grade. If the proposals are accepted, all new doctors will enter a two-year foundation programme that includes the current pre-registration year, to help them develop core skills and sample a range of practice settings. A time-limited specialist training programme will follow this. Both types of programme will have defined curricula, entry requirements and assessments, all of which will be managed by the postgraduate deans of medical schools (DoH 2002a).

The British Medical Association estimates that there are approximately 20,000 senior house officers in the UK (BMA 2002). These junior doctors perform much of the day-to-day work with patients. The proposed changes raise questions about whether they will continue to do so and who will fill any ensuing gaps in service. Past experience is not encouraging on this point in that the nurse practitioner roles were introduced in the early 1990s in response to changes in the working conditions for doctors. It is to be anticipated that nurses will once again be expected to make up the shortfall in service provision.

Aside from the issue of junior doctors' hours, staff shortages are a perennial problem. The NHS Plan stated that these would be improved using multiple strategies that included raising the numbers of places on training courses and encouraging former health professionals, especially nurses, to return to practice (DoH 2000). Inevitably, the projected figures will take time, years in fact, to achieve. This situation creates both opportunities and challenges for advanced practice. In terms of opportunities, advanced practitioners have the chance to demonstrate their effectiveness and the contribution that they can make to patient care. Menard (1987) argues that one of the triggers for acceptance of advanced practice in the USA was staff shortages in civilian hospitals during World War II and the Korean and Vietnam wars. Civilian nurses found themselves responsible for critically ill patients and developed skills to meet their needs. Their military counterparts in field hospitals had the opportunity to care for critically wounded patients who survived because of improvements in technology. In peacetime, the changes that had occurred could not be reversed and there were sufficient numbers of nurses with the new expertise to create a critical mass and thus a force for change. The challenge for those nurses was the same as that facing advanced practitioners in the UK: that is, to ensure that change takes place within the scope of nursing and does not become a covert way of producing more doctors or medical technicians.

We therefore recommend that those responsible for developing and managing advanced posts retain a focus on nursing. Whilst the intention of advanced practice is to adjust the boundaries of nursing by exploring new possibilities, this does not mean that nurses can replace another profession. Arguments that nurses are cheaper to employ than doctors are unlikely to be successful given that the proposals for pay reform focus on the evaluation of jobs: a nurse expected to take the same responsibilities as a doctor would, therefore, cost the same to employ. We also recommend that advanced practice posts are subject to regular review and that any decisions about pay and job evaluation take account of the experimental dimensions of developing new roles. It may be that advanced practitioners who in time become well established in their posts will be able to act as consultants in guiding the introduction of new jobs alongside the more traditional expertise offered by unions and staff organisations. Finally we emphasise the importance of professional cohesion to lobby for recognition of advanced practitioners and to provide support for individuals as they continue to lead nursing forward.

Advanced practice and first contact services

The NHS Plan made a commitment to increasing access to healthcare by ensuring that all patients would be able to see a health professional in primary care within 24 hours and a GP within two days (DoH 2000). The nursing strategy that accompanied the Plan made clear that nurses had a key role to play in achieving such targets and ensuring that services are appropriately responsive to patients' needs (DoH 1999).

One proposal arising from this is the development of first contact services. It is envisaged that community nurses, and potentially other community-based practitioners such as pharmacists, who have received additional preparation in pathophysiology, advanced health assessment, primary care leadership and management, will become the first point of contact for patients. These nurses will assess patients, advise on self-care or initiate treatment, referring to the GP only those with complex needs.

Training for this role will be based in the workplace. Individuals will be asked to complete a self-assessment tool to establish their suitability for entry to the programme and accredit prior learning. Once accepted, students will be expected to take responsibility for their own learning under the guidance of a clinical education manager. Assessment will focus on determining individual ability to accurately assess and diagnose. The training will be managed through the National Health Service University in partnership with primary care trusts and will be set at MSc level.

The idea of first contact services is at present intended only for England. Primary care trusts and practitioners will be canvassed to determine learning needs and map current programmes. There are ten pilot sites in different parts of the country and work is under way on developing self-assessment tools, distance learning materials and software. Expansion of the programme will begin in summer 2004 if the pilot evaluates successfully.

The concept of first contact services is compatible with that of advanced practice. The criteria published by the International Council of Nurses (see page 147) clearly states that advanced practitioners have expanded clinical competences that enable them to act as first contact providers of healthcare (ICN 2002). In many settings they may be the only provider available. The World Health Organisation has recommended that health service providers take account of this and become more flexible and creative, identifying new approaches that meet the needs of local populations, particularly the poor, socially excluded, isolated or marginalised, rather than continue to rely on outmoded custom and practice (WHO 2000). Advanced practice can, therefore, be regarded as part of the front-line healthcare services. The advanced practitioner is qualified to apply nursing knowledge and skill to meet the everyday healthcare needs of patients, referring them to a doctor or other health professional only when that knowledge and skill are exceeded by patient needs (Smith 1995). The first contact service proposed for the UK takes a similar view, that first contact professionals should be able to meet the healthcare needs of about 70% of all patients, thus leaving medical staff more time to devote to those who need their unique skills (DoH 2002b; Ions 2002). We therefore recommend that advanced practitioners give serious consideration to the first contact service proposal and explore ways in which they may be able to apply their expertise.

The future of advanced practice in the UK

We anticipate that advanced practice will continue to evolve to provide articulate and creative professional leadership. Inherent in this leadership will be the need to

- Explore participative approaches to patient care based on true partnerships so that the delivery of care becomes a process of *doing with* rather than *doing to* others
- Clarify speciality-based competences that, when combined with the national standard developed by the UKCC, create a comprehensive picture of advanced roles in diverse settings
- Critically examine the methodological issues in evaluating the impact and effectiveness of advanced practice and develop creative approaches to establishing and testing patient oriented criteria
- Develop collaborative working relationships with medical colleagues and work constructively to overcome barriers to the acceptance of advanced practice in healthcare.

We anticipate that advanced practitioners will continue to seek out ways of improving care for patients and respond creatively to the challenges ahead. We wish them well.

? **Exercise for evaluating websites**

Select a specific problem area of relevance to your work. This may be a clinical problem such as a particular condition experienced by your patient/client group, a functional problem such as incontinence, or some other issue arising, for example management, training or education.

Identify **three** websites that deal with this problem area.

Critically appraise each of these sites, taking into account the following:

- Whom the site is intended for. Ideally you should try to identify sites aimed at different groups. For example, sites about diabetes may be aimed at patients/relatives/doctors, etc. Some sites may reflect a particular point of view: for example, some organisations may concentrate on lobbying for a certain type of treatment or emphasise self-help.
- The overall quality of the information that each provides, whether it is evidence-based and the possible usefulness of it in your practice.
- The treatments and interventions listed and whether these are available in the NHS.
- Ease of location and use.
- When each site was last updated.
- Links to other sites.
- The advice you would give to patients/carers/relatives/colleagues about this site.

References

BMA (2002) *BMA Response to Consultation on Unfinished Business.* Available at http://www.bma.org.uk

DoH (1999) *Making a Difference: Strengthening the Nursing, Midwifery and Health Visiting Contribution to Health and Healthcare.* London: DoH.

DoH (2000) *The NHS Plan: A Plan for Investment, A Plan for Reform.* London: DoH.

DoH (2001) *Implementing the NHS Plan: Modern Matrons. Strengthening the Role of Ward Sisters and Introducing Senior Sisters,* Health Service Circular 2001/10. Available at http://www.doh.gov.uk/hsc.htm

DoH (2002a) *Unfinished Business: Proposals for the Reform of the Senior House Officer Grade. Report by Sir Liam Donaldson. A paper for consultation.* Available at http://www.doh.gov.uk

DoH (2002b) Chief nursing officer's report. Available at http://www.doh.gov.uk

Hamric, A. (2000) A definition of advanced nursing practice. In *Advanced Nursing Practice: An Integrative Approach,* 2nd edn (eds A. Hamric, J. Spross & C. Hanson), pp. 53–73. Philadelphia: W.B. Saunders.

Hunsberger, M., Mitchell, A., Blatz, S., Paes, B., Pinelli, J., Southwell, D., French, S. & Soluk, R. (1992) Definition of an advanced nursing practice role in the NICU: the clinical nurse specialist/neonatal practitioner. *Clinical Nurse Specialist,* 6 (2): 91–6.

ICN (2002) http://icn.org (accessed September 2002).

Ions, V. (2002) Delivering quality access services in primary care: supporting the role of the nurse providing first contact services programme. Unpublished briefing paper. London: DoH.

Koetters, T. (1989) Clinical practice and direct patient care. In: *The Clinical Nurse Specialist in Theory and Practice,* 2nd edn (eds A. Hamric & J. Spross), pp. 107–24, Philadelphia: W.B. Saunders.

Marriner-Tomey, A. (1993) *Transformational Leadership in Nursing.* St Louis: Mosby.

Menard, S. (ed.) (1987) *The Clinical Nurse Specialist: Perspectives on Practice.* New York: John Wiley.

NHS (1999) *Agenda for Change: Modernising the NHS Pay System. Joint framework of Principles and Agreed Statement on the Way Forward,* HSC 1999/227. Available at http://www.doh.gov.uk

Sackett, D.L., Richardson, W.S., Muir, J.A. Haynes, R.B. & Richardson, W.S. (1996) Evidence-based medicine: what it is and what it isn't. *British Medical Journal,* 312 (13): 71–2.

Shay, L., Goldstein, J., Matthews, D., Trail, L. & Edmunds, M. (1996) Guidelines for developing a nurse practitioner practice. *Nurse Practitioner,* 21 (1): 74–6, 78, 81.

Smith, M. (1995) The core of advanced nursing practice. *Nursing Science Quarterly,* 8 (1): 2–3.

UKCC (2002) *Report of the Higher Level of Practice Pilot and Project.* London: UKCC.

WHO (2000) *Global Advisory Group on Nursing and Midwifery. Report of the 6th Meeting.* Geneva: WHO. Available at www.who.org (accessed September 2002).

Index